Olimpio Rodríguez Santos
Enrique Toribio Pájaro
Roberto Galeana Ríos

Respiratory and digestive tract diseases with sleep apnea

Olimpio Rodríguez Santos
Enrique Toribio Pájaro
Roberto Galeana Ríos

Respiratory and digestive tract diseases with sleep apnea

Interdisciplinary approach

ScienciaScripts

Imprint

Any brand names and product names mentioned in this book are subject to trademark, brand or patent protection and are trademarks or registered trademarks of their respective holders. The use of brand names, product names, common names, trade names, product descriptions etc. even without a particular marking in this work is in no way to be construed to mean that such names may be regarded as unrestricted in respect of trademark and brand protection legislation and could thus be used by anyone.

Cover image: www.ingimage.com

This book is a translation from the original published under ISBN 978-620-3-03447-9.

Publisher:
Sciencia Scripts
is a trademark of
Dodo Books Indian Ocean Ltd. and OmniScriptum S.R.L publishing group

120 High Road, East Finchley, London, N2 9ED, United Kingdom
Str. Armeneasca 28/1, office 1, Chisinau MD-2012, Republic of Moldova, Europe
Managing Directors: Ieva Konstantinova, Victoria Ursu
info@omniscriptum.com

Printed at: see last page
ISBN: 978-620-4-08166-3

Copyright © Olimpio Rodríguez Santos, Enrique Toribio Pájaro, Roberto Galeana Ríos
Copyright © 2021 Dodo Books Indian Ocean Ltd. and OmniScriptum S.R.L publishing group

Respiratory and digestive tract diseases associated with sleep disorders. Interdisciplinary approach

Dr. Olimpio Rodriguez Santos
Dr.C. Valentin Santiago Rodriguez Moya
Dr. Edilberto Machado del Risco.
Dr. Enrique Toribio Pajaro
Dr. Roberto Galeana Rios
Dr. Raul Alberto Rojas Galarza
Dr. Cristian Ponce Alvarez
Dr. Gabriela Jardines Arciniega
Dr. Ricardo Olea Zapata
Dr. Nora Elizabeth Vite Juarez
Zuriel Flores Silverio

Contents

Introduction 5
Chapter 1 9
Chapter 2 30
Chapter 3 44
Chapter 4 49
Chapter 5 75
Chapter 6 86
Chapter 7 126

Authors

Dr. Olimpio Rodriguez Santos
Doctor of Medicine, Havana 1979. Specialist of I and II Degree in Allergology, Havana 1985 and 2003. Master in Medical Humanities and Higher Education. Assistant Professor of the universities of Camaguey. Auxiliary Researcher Ministry of Culture. Publications: articles, 76. Books, 9. Referee of several Biomedical journals. Honorary member of the College of Physicians and Surgeons of Cuautla, Mexico. E-Mail: olimpio49@gmail.com

Dr.C. Valentin Santiago Rodriguez Moya
Doctor of Medicine, Medical University of Camaguey "Dr. Carlos J. Finlay, 1997 Specialist of first degree in Pediatrics, 2002. First degree specialist in Intensive Care and Pediatric Emergencies, 2009 and 2014. Assistant Professor and researcher at the University of Medical Sciences "Carlos J. Finlay" 2016 and 2017. Doctor of Medical Sciences awarded by the Ministry of Higher Education of the Republic of Cuba.

Dr. Edilberto Machado del Risco.
Doctor of Medicine. First Degree Specialist in Allergology 1997. Second Degree Specialist in Allergology 2010. Assistant Professor 2013. Head of the Provincial Group of Allergy in Camaguey. Expert of the specialty designated by the Minsap. Publications: 14. Arbitration of biomedical journals: Vaccimonitor and Gaceta Medica Espirituana. Affiliation to the Cuban Society of Allergy, Asthma and Clinical Immunology. Member of the World Allergy Organization. Honorary member of the College of Physicians and Surgeons of Cuautla, Mexico.

Dr. Enrique Toribio Pajaro
Surgeon and midwife from BUAP, 1973. Specialist in Pediatrics, 1981 at the National Institute of Pediatrics. Specialist in Infectology, 1985, National School of Biological Sciences. Specialist in Clinical Immunology and Allergies, 1993 at the IPN. E-Mail: drenriquetoribio@hotmail.com

Dr. Roberto Galeana Rios
Surgeon, Faculty of Medicine, Autonomous University of Guerrero 2006.
Diploma in Allergology 2009 and Diploma in Immunotherapy of allergy in children under 5 years Policlfnico Previsora Camaguey Cuba.2018. Advanced Immunology Course IPN. National School of Biological Sciences 2011. Diploma in Diagnostic Endoscopy UAGro 2011. Resident of Allergy and Clinical Immunology (AAIBA) 2020. Email: garios07@hotmail.com

Dr. Raul Alberto Rojas Galarza
Physician, Specialist in Pediatrics. Subspecialist in Gastroenterology. Pediatrics. Master in Public Health. Professional Specialist in Implementation and Audit of Integrated Quality Management Systems, Environment,

Risk Management and Corrective Action Management. Medical Auditor. Specialist in Occupational Health and Safety at Work. Member of the *Critical Appraisal Skills Programme* (CASP) Peru. Cochrane Reviewer. Teacher at the Peruvian University of Applied Sciences (UPC), Lima Peru. Pediatrician at the National Institute of Child Health (INSN), Lima Peru. Pediatric Gastroenterologist at the 'Carita Feliz' Clinic, Piura Peru. Researcher and author of national and international publications.

Dr. Cristian Ponce Alvarez
Surgeon and midwife, National Polytechnic Institute, 2007. Update on the diagnosis and treatment of severe anaphylactic reaction, San Diego Medical Center, 2008. Update in the diagnosis and treatment of near lethal asthma, Centro Medico San Diego, 2008. Diploma in Allergology, 2013. Diploma in Immunotherapy of allergy in children under 5 years 2017, Policlfnico Previsora Camaguey Cuba. Resident of Allergy and Clinical Immunology (AAIBA) 2020. Email: dr.cristian.ponce@hotmail.com.

Dr. Gabriela Jardines Arciniega.
Surgeon and midwife, National Polytechnic Institute, 2009. Diploma in Allergology, 2013. Resident of Allergy and Clinical Immunology (AAIBA) 2020. Participation in the observational study of obstructive pulmonary disease (NOVELTY), AstraZeneca AB, Argentina.
Email: drajag@hotmail.com.

Dr. Ricardo Olea Zapata
Surgeon 1995 National University of Piura. Postgraduate School of the National University of Piura. Master in University Teaching 2005. UNMSM Title of Pediatrician. Medical College of Peru. Collegiate N° 29104, 1,995. Medical College of Peru. Post degree. Residency in the specialty of Pediatrics. Institute of Child Health. UNMSM. June 1997- May 2000. Peruvian Society of Pediatrics Piura Branch - full member since June 2002 E-mail riolza1@hotmail.com

Dr. Nora Elizabeth Vite Juarez
Surgeon 1995 National University of Piura. Postgraduate School of the National University of Piura Master in University Teaching 2005. UNMSM. Title of Pediatrician Medical College of Peru. Collegiate N° 29104, 1,995. Medical College of Peru. Residency in the specialty of Pediatrics: Institute of Child Health. UNMSM. June 1997- May 2000. Peruvian Society of Pediatrics Piura Branch. Full member since June 2002.
E-mail: noravitejuarez@hotmail.com.pe

Zuriel Flores Silverio
Student UNAM. Faculty of Higher Studies Zaragoza. Researcher on behalf of the UNAM FES Zaragoza zurel98@gmail.com

Introduction

Respiratory and digestive tract diseases associated with sleep disorders. Interdisciplinary approach, is a manual whose authors approach us to a text directed, fundamentally, towards primary health care (PHC). However, the content goes beyond PHC, since many of its authors are professionals whose vision of the problem corresponds to other levels of health and have also been through PHC, so that the objective of the work remains latent. Some of these professionals have gained their experience in private clinics or public hospitals, including pediatric intensive care units. For this reason, they have given the contents the necessary depth to be useful to general practitioners and specialists at all levels of health who are dedicated to the care of patients suffering from allergic diseases, asthma and esophagitis.

Allergy and asthma are effects of an inappropriate immune response, often to common allergens such as mites, pollen, fungi, food or animal dander. The possibility that certain substances increase sensitivity in vertebrates rather than protect them was recognized by Charles Richet as early as 1902. It happened when he tried to immunize dogs against the toxins of a type of jellyfish called *Physalia*.

Richet and Paul Portier noted that dogs exposed to sub-lethal doses of the toxin reacted almost instantly and fatally to further contact with very small amounts of the same toxin. Richet concluded that successful immunization or vaccination created *phyllaxis,* or protection, and that the opposite result, anaphylaxis, could be observed, in which exposure to the anUgen could precipitate a potentially lethal sensitivity if the exposure were repeated. Thus revealing the anaphylactic reaction for which he received the Nobel Prize in 1913.

The current increase in sensitization, due to repeated contact with environmental allergens, is the cause of the increase in anaphylaxis in most countries. This results in an increase in allergic diseases and asthma. Allergic rhinitis (AR) has the highest incidence. It has been shown that 52.8% of adults with AR have poor sleep quality and 21.1% suffer from excessive daytime sleepiness. People with asthma are also at increased risk for sleep apnea, and may wake up during the night due to the symptoms of this disorder.

Similarly, nocturnal reflux esophagitis and other types of esophagitis frequently affect individuals with sleep apnea, so the presence of sleep disorder associated with these diseases, invites further study, seeking a better quality of life in this population group. This involves studying those diseases of the upper respiratory and digestive tract in which sleep apnea may be involved, specifying the symptoms of each one.

The symptoms of erosive esophagitis depend on the degree of esophageal injury. The most common are vomiting with or without blood, pain when eating solid foods or consuming liquids, blood in the stool, sore throat, hoarseness, chest pain and chronic cough.

Erosive esophagitis is a serious condition and when it is not treated properly, it can cause anemia due to lack of iron, in the most severe cases, the appearance of a tumor in the esophagus. Therefore, if there is suspicion of this condition, it is essential to go to the Gastroenterologist so that the diagnosis can be made and treatment can be initiated. The diagnosis of erosive esophagitis is made by evaluating the symptoms presented and the factors that improve or worsen their intensity. Erosive esophagitis occurs when lesions form in the esophagus due to chronic gastroesophageal reflux. Cases of erosive esophagitis can be the most severe form of common esophagitis, which ended up developing lesions because it was not treated correctly. The treatment of this condition is usually indicated by the Gastroenterologist, who may recommend the use of medications to avoid the excess of gastric juice or even inhibit its production; on the other hand, in the most severe situations, surgery may be suggested. It is also necessary to be followed by a nutritionist, in order to indicate which are the alterations to be made in the habits. Proton pump inhibitors (PPIs), such as omeprazole, esomeprazole and lansoprazole, which inhibit the production of gastric juice by the stomach, preventing it from reaching the esophagus, should be used; histamine H2-receptor inhibitors, such as ranitidine, famotidine, cimetidine and nizatidine; used when PPIs do not produce the expected effect, helping to reduce the amount of acid in the stomach; procinetics, such as domperidone and metoclopramide; used to accelerate the emptying of the stomach.

In case the person is under treatment with anticholinergics, such as Artane or Akineton, or calcium channel blockers, such as amlodipine or verapamil, the Gastroenterologist can give specific recommendations on how to use the prescribed medications. Surgery for erosive esophagitis is only indicated if the lesions do not improve or when symptoms are persistent and all of the above treatment options have been used. This surgery consists of reconstructing a small valve that separates the junction between the esophagus and the stomach, thus preventing gastric juice from flowing back through the esophagus and causing new lesions.

The purpose of this book is that professionals who are dedicated to the management of allergy and asthma also take into account the symptomatology and treatment of esophagitis and, above all, that they can identify the sleep disorders that can occur in all of them, always looking for an expanded horizontal view to strengthen the quality of life of this large group of patients.

In the first chapter, the basic immunology is presented with details about the immune response (IR) and its main components. In the following chapters, each of the aforementioned diseases is discussed in more detail.

Bibliography

Aronson JK. Proton pump inhibitors. In: Aronson JK, ed. *Meyers Side Effects of Drugs*. 16th ed. Walthman, MA: Elsevier; 2016:1040-1045.

Sleep apnea and nocturnal reflux esophagitis. *Archives of Internal Medicine 2003; 163:41-45* http://archinte.ama-assn.org/

Leoz G. One hundred years of anaphylaxis and allergy. Arch Soc Esp Oftalmol [Internet]. 2003 Jan [cited 2020 Dec 29]; 78(1): 59-60. Available at: http://scielo.isciii.es/scielo.php?script=sciarttext&pid=S0365-66912003003000100014&lng=en

Richter JE, Friedenberg FK. Gastroesophageal reflux disease. In: Feldman M, Friedman LS, Brandt LJ, eds. *Sleisenger and Fordtran's Gastrointestinal and Liver Disease*. 10th ed. Philadelphia, PA: Elsevier Saunders; 2016:chap 44.

Chapter 1
Basic immunology to address allergic diseases, asthma and other conditions.

Dr. Olimpio Rodnguez Santos, Dr. Enrique Toribio Pajaro, Dr. Ricardo Olea Zapata, Dra. Nora Elizabeth Vite Juarez

The immunology developed in the book deals with the innate immune system (IBS), with its physical and chemical barriers, cells, blood proteins and cytokines. In the same sense it refers to the IR, being, the acquired immune response (AIR) predominantly humoral, cellular and mixed. When immunity is acquired, the response can be active natural, such as infection, or artificial in vaccines, and passive natural, if it is transferred from another subject, as occurs from mother to fetus and child, and artificial by gamma globulins. Depending on the number of required contacts with the anUgen, IR can be primary or secondary.

The three most important cells of the immune system (IS) are the dendritic cells (DCs) - innate and presenters to viral T-lymphocytes, T-lymphocytes (orchestrators of RIA, helpers of B and effectors against intracellular pathogens) and B-lymphocytes (producers of antibodies, effectors against extracellular pathogens).

The remarkable facts of RIA are specificity, self tolerance, diversity, clonal expansion, immunopolarization, contraction, homeostasis and immune memory. There are five phases of RIA: recognition, activation (expansion and differentiation), elimination, contraction and memory.

The antigen recognition molecules of the innate immune response (IAR) are three: the pattern recognition receptors (PRR) and the class II and class I antigen presenting molecules (APM). Those of the IAR are two: the T-lymphocyte receptor (TCR) and the B-lymphocyte receptor (BCR).

Foreign substances can be classified, according to their ability to induce RIA or not, into immunogens, anUgens and haptens; by their origin into autoanUgens, isoanUgens, alloanUgens or xenoanUgens; by their nature into proteins, carbohydrates, kpids and nucleic acids; and, by their spatial structure into linear or conformational.

The immunogenicity or ability to induce an IR is determined by the character of the foreign, its chemical nature, its size, its complexity, the genetic constitution of the host, the route of administration, the dose, the frequency and the use of adjuvants.

In humans, the antibody classes IgM, IgG, IgA, IgE and IgD (DAMEG, as a mnemotechnical resource) are produced, consisting of two heavy chains, where the differences between them reside, and two light chains, which in turn have a constant and a variable portion. The antibodies allow the antigen-antibody interaction through non-covalent interactions where their specificity is their main property.

The anticipated repertoire of TCRs and BCRs occurs, in the absence of anUgens, by a similar somatic recombination process in both receptors. However, after antigenic recognition, only the BCR amplifies its repertoire due to two processes: somatic hypermutation or affinity maturation and class switching or isotype switching.

The TCR always remains bound to the T lymphocyte so its action is local. However, the BCR can be bound to the B lymphocyte as a monomeric IgM receptor or the lymphocyte can transform into a plasma cell and initially secrete pentameric soluble IgM, so that the antibody can act locally and at a distance. This occurs by alternative processing at the level of primary RNA transcription. The TCR and BCR are expressed only on T and B lymphocytes, respectively. Class II MPPs are expressed on peptide-presenting cells (dendritic cells, macrophages and activated B cells); but only DCs present peptides to v^gene T cells. Macrophages and B-lymphocytes also do so, but in the effector phase. Class I MPPs present in all nucleated cells and platelets present peptides to TCD8; but mainly in the effector phase of IR.

Lymphoid organs are classified as primary (bone marrow and thymus), secondary (Waldeyer's ring, lymph nodes, spleen, Peyer's patches and appendix) and tertiary (neoformed). In the primary lymphocytes are produced and in the secondary lymphocytes the IR is orchestrated.

The IS of vertebrates and humans, consists of various organs and different cells, which allow the organism to distinguish its own and eliminate the foreign, with the consequent protection against diseases, developing immunity. Immunity derives from the Latin word *immunitas,* which refers to the protection of the immune system.

immunity from legal process enjoyed by Roman senators while in office. However, the term immunity nowadays refers to protection against infectious diseases. The thymus and bone marrow (Fig. 1 and 2) are the primary organs of the IS. The thymus resembles the endocrine glands, not only because it develops from the third brachial arch, but also because it has the structure of an internal secretion gland. It has been conferred a central role in the development of the cellular IS, being responsible for the development and maturation of T lymphocytes. The function of the thymus is exerted primarily through the hormones thymosins. The function of the organ is exerted, predominantly in neonates and in children, and regresses after puberty, when the main lymphoid tissues are destroyed.

are fully developed.

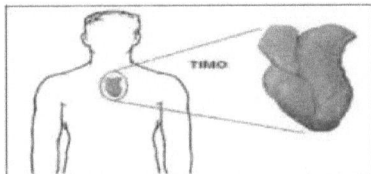 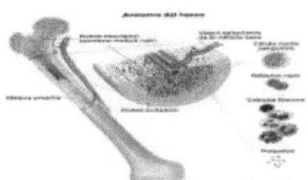

Fig. 1. Thymus.

Fig. 2. Bone marrow. Anatomy of the

Bone marrow is the spongy tissue found inside bones, such as in the hip and thigh bones. It contains stem cells that can grow into red blood cells to carry oxygen, white blood cells that fight infection, and platelets that help blood clot. When there is bone marrow disease, there are problems with the stem cells or with their development as in leukemia, aplastic anemia and myeloproliferative diseases. Leukemia is a blood cancer, where the bone marrow produces abnormal white blood cells. In aplastic anemia, the bone marrow does not produce red blood cells.

In myeloproliferative diseases, the bone marrow produces too many white blood cells. Other diseases such as lymphoma can spread to the bone marrow and affect the production of blood cells. Causes of bone marrow diseases include genetic and environmental factors. Tests include blood and bone marrow tests. Treatments depend on the disorder and its severity. They may involve medications, blood transfusions, or a bone marrow transplant.

The cells and molecules responsible for immunity constitute the structure of the IS. The joint and coordinated response of the IS, when foreign substances are introduced into the body, is called the immune response (IR). In the particular case of people suffering from allergic diseases, they present a characteristic type of IR as we will see below.

The bone marrow generates B-lymphocytes and T-precursors, matures B-lymphocytes v^genes and stores memory lymphocytes.

In the thymus T precursors mature and the processes of MPP restriction and tolerization occur. Restriction occurs by positive selection where only lymphocytes that recognize their own MPPs survive. Tolerization occurs by negative selection where lymphocytes that recognize self-antigens with high affinity are eliminated.

Orchestration of IR leads to proliferation and clonal differentiation of T and B lymphocytes in secondary lymphoid organs. The antigen presenting cells are DCs, macrophages and activated B-lymphocytes presenting peptides in MPP-II. However, DCs are the real professionals for the stimulation of T-lymphocyte viruses. All nucleated cells and platelets present peptides at MPP-I. B and T lymphocytes are the only cells in the body that recirculate and patrol the body against aggressors. All leukocytes including lymphocytes can be extravasated by rolling, stopping and migrating into tissues.

The stages of maturation of B lymphocytes in the bone marrow are: Pro-B, PreB (early and late) and immature. They complete their maturation in the periphery. B lymphocytes are subdivided into conventional B-2 and B-1, belonging to the RIA and RII, respectively. B-1 lymphocytes predominate in the fetus, neonate and adult tissues, recognize particularly polysaccharides, preferentially induce IgM and no immune memory, and are self-renewing and therefore long-lived.

B lymphocytes are dominated by central negative selection, as they use IgM as a BCR and do not require MPP to recognize antigens. For positive selection they require the help of T lymphocytes to switch to plasmacytes.

The mechanisms of central tolerance at the B level are clonal deletion, anergy and Treg. Immune tolerance is a specific non-responsive RIA with memory against the inducer called tolerogen. It can affect either of the two RIA populations, T and B lymphocytes or both. It can also occur centrally or peripherally.

According to the mechanisms of production, immune tolerance can be by deletion, anergy or suppression. Deletion is the mechanism of immune tolerance that consists in the total elimination of the organism of the tolerized cells, a process that occurs by apoptosis. Clonal anergy is the immune tolerance mechanism that silences B and T lymphocytes without their physical elimination.

The physical factors of the barriers are: mucus, glycocalyx, desmosomes, intestinal peristaltic movements, airway cilia and commensal microbiota.

The presence of PRR to recognize microbial-associated molecular patterns (MAMP) and damage-associated molecular patterns (DAMP) is designed to reduce inflammation and thus reduce mucosal damage. Thus, the Toll-like receptor (TLR-4) that recognizes the potent endotoxin lipopolysaccharide (LPS) of Gram- bacteria is decreased in the luminal region and lacks its co-receptor CD14.

Commensals are involved in the formation of germinal centers (B lymphocyte activity) in newborns and in maintaining mucosal homeostasis. Acquired immune defenses are constituted by T and B lymphocytes and IgAS. IgAS is the main mucosal protective antibody and the one that is produced in the greatest quantity in humans. The mechanisms by which IgAS functions are immune exclusion, viral neutralization, toxin neutralization and immune clearance.

IgG, which also protects mucous membranes, is passively transferred by diffusion when its blood concentrations are high.

Vaccines and immunity

In order to maintain and improve immunity, throughout history man has created vaccines. They have eliminated or reduced important infectious diseases that are scourges for humanity, causing the loss of millions of lives or causing irreversible disorders. Among them are smallpox, measles, rubella, bacterial meningoencephalitis, diphtheria, tetanus and poliomyelitis. These vaccines use weakened or dead germs such as viruses or bacteria to initiate IR in the body.

Research is also continuing on the development of vaccines for different types of cancer that are a hard blow to humanity. These vaccines can be preventive and therapeutic. Preventive vaccines are for some types of cancer caused by viruses. Vaccines that help protect against infection with these viruses may also help prevent some of these cancers. Some strains of human papillomavirus (HPV) have been linked to cancers of the cervix, anus, throat, vagina, vulva, and penis. In fact, most cervical cancers are caused by HPV infection. Vaccinating children, certain teens and adults against HPV helps protect against cervical cancer and five other types of cancer.

People who have chronic hepatitis B virus (HBV) infections have an increased risk of liver cancer. Getting the vaccine to help prevent HBV infection may reduce the risk of liver cancer.

These are traditional preventive vaccines that target viruses that can cause certain types of cancer. They may help protect against some types of cancer, but they do not directly target cancer cells because cancer cells have not yet formed or been found.

These types of vaccines are useful for cancers caused by infection. However, most cancers, such as colorectal, lung, prostate, and breast cancers, are not thought to be caused by infections.

Therapeutic vaccines to treat cancer are different from vaccines that work against viruses in that they try to prime the IS to launch an attack against cancer cells in the body. These vaccines aim to get the IS to attack a disease that already exists.

Some cancer treatment vaccines are made up of cancer cells, parts of cells, or pure anUgens such as certain proteins in cancer cells. Sometimes a patient's own immune cells are removed and exposed to these substances in the laboratory to create the vaccine. Once the vaccine is ready, it is injected into the body to increase the IR against the cancer cells.

Vaccines are often combined with other substances or cells called *adjuvants* that help to further increase RI.

Cancer vaccines cause the IS to attack cells with one or more specific antigens. Because the IS has special immune memory cells, it is expected that the vaccine can continue to work long after it is given.

Despite the enormous benefit of prophylactic and therapeutic vaccines, the best protection against infectious agents occurs when the human being recovers from a natural infection, infections that generally occur in childhood. This better protection depends on several factors. Among them, the infection occurs with a living organism that exposes all of its immune components to the infection and when the infection is eliminated, it is because the organism has identified the vital substances of the pathogen and has elaborated effective responses against them.

Therapeutic vaccines also include allergy vaccines, which are often referred to as allergen-specific immunotherapy (ASIT). When a small amount of the allergen is injected into the body or applied to the mucous membranes, the IS produces a substance called an antibody that prevents the allergen from causing the symptoms characteristic of allergic diseases.

Mucosal immune system

The mucosa represents the main immune tissue of the organism with about 400 m^2, 222 times greater than the skin, which has an approximate area of 1.8 m^2, so it must defend us from more than 90% of human infections. The 90% of the cells of the organism is constituted by microbiota, predominating in the colon. More than 95% of the infections arrive or settle in the mucous membranes.

The human has about 10^{13} cells which amounts to 10 million million million cells. In the intestine alone there are 10 times more (10^{14}) commensal and pathogenic bacteria of about 1500 different species. In the colon there are about 10^{11}-10^{12} bacteria per g of feces of about 500 commensal species. In the neo are about 10^8 pathogenic bacteria per mL. In the mouth there are about 200 pathogenic species. In the stomach with its drastic pH changes it is present in up to 50 % of the population.

Conservative estimates suggest that more than 50% of the world's population has a stomach colonized by Helicobacter pylori, a gram-negative, helical bacillus-like bacterium that inhabits the human gastric epithelium. Infection by H. pylori can cause inflammation of the gastric mucosa leading to gastritis, peptic ulcer and mucosa-associated lymphoid tissue lymphoma. 90% of the human organism is made up of exogenous cells. Thus, we can become ill with internal pathogens if our immune defenses that keep them in check are lowered, as in the case of immunosuppression that can be produced by sustained stress. Also by being healthy carriers we can spread infections to susceptible people. These people without signs or symptoms of disease, but infected, are carriers, constituting the main epidemiological risk for the transmission of diseases. In cases of immunodeficiency some commensals may also become pathogenic. Consequently, the mucosal system must have strong innate and acquired defences to control these pathogens and commensals on a huge and very vulnerable surface.

The mucosal IS has to develop, simultaneously, contrasting IR, in order to be able to differentiate food from commensals and especially from pathogens.

In the main mucosal tissues there are inductor and effector sites. Inducer sites contain Peyer's patches that allow the sampling of particulate antigens and effector sites are located in the submucosa.

The only professional antigen-presenting cell, to the T-lymphocytes, is the DCs that are sentinel cells in the tissues and travel to the secondary lymphoid organs. Immature DCs in the periphery migrate within hours as they mature to secondary lymphoid organs where IR is orchestrated.

DCs acquire the anUgens, the extracellular or exogenous and intracellular or endogenous forms. These are degraded and presented in the MPP-II or MPP-I, respectively. There is also cross-presentation.

The activation of B-lymphocytes depends on whether the antigen is thymus-dependent (activates B-1) or thymodependent (activates B-2). Only B-2 require T-helper.

Cell cooperation is the process through which IS cells interact for the induction of IR and the production of its effectors. Particularly important are the interaction: CD-TCD4 v^genes, TCD4-macrophage, TCD4-B and TCD4-TCD8. Effective cooperation between CD-TCD4 v^genes in secondary lymphoid organs requires close and stable contact between the two cells, a process known as immunological synapse.

Five laws govern RII and RIA: the promptness of the response (occurrence); the molecules used, their specificities, their diversities and the recall of previous contacts or memory.

RII is phylogenetically conserved, has its mediators in all cells, recognizes danger signals, involves less than 100 components, is less limited, detects pathogen species, does not recognize cryptic or altered peptides and few failures occur. RIA appears in vertebrates, its mediators only in T and B lymphocytes and their derivatives, distinguishes self from non-self, is self-limited, detects soluble antigens or peptides, detects exogens and altered self, and has more frequent failures than RII.

The physical barriers are constituted by the skin and mucous membranes. Molecular barriers are made up of cytokines and complement. Cytokines are intercellular communication molecules secreted by various cells of the RII and RIA. Complement is a system of more than 30 serum proteins.

Cytokines function in autocrine, paracrine, pleiotropic, redundant, synergistic, endocrine and inhibitory ways. Cytokines can also be classified according to their effects: proinflammatory; growth factors; polarizing towards Th1 or Th2 responses and inhibitory. Cytokines can be classified according to the extracellular and intracellular homologues of their receptors: haemopoietin;

chemokines and families of IL1 and TNF.

The Complement system is a set of more than 30 serum proteins that make up the classical, alternative and lectin systems. Complement by any of its active pathways directly lyses pathogens, including opsonins (C3b and C4b) and anaphyllotoxins. It works by producing efficient lysis of pathogens, production of anaphyllotoxins and kinins, opsonization, activation of B-lymphocytes, bactericidal effect and solubilization of immunocomplexes.

The dynamics of IR is a law present throughout the development of IR that is dependent on the pathogen, its gateway and host genetic factors.

Pathogens can be grouped into intracellular, where acquired protective responses are mediated mainly by cytotoxic T lymphocytes (CTL) and extracellular where antibodies are the most effective including IgE against helminths.

Helminths establish chronic infestations requiring amplification of innate defense mechanisms (basophils, mast cells and eosinophils) by acquired ones (Th2 and IgE). While many viruses, bacteria and protozoa produce acute infections that are won only by the innate response.

The placental mucosa requires a separate dynamic approach as uterine NKs predominate. The cytokines produced change during pregnancy; there are other suppressive factors and there may be particular infections in the placenta.

The dynamics of RIA include: lymphocyte recirculation, T-cell support, primary and secondary antibody response. The categories of RIA are latency, intensity, duration and memory.

Endocytosis of large solid particles is called phagocytosis, when they are soluble it is called pinocytosis and they can be opsonized by facilitating entry through receptors.

The main phagocytes are neutrophils and macrophages. Neutrophils originate in the bone marrow and migrate into the blood, entering the tissues under conditions of inflammation, while monocytes, which also originate in the bone marrow, exit into the blood, but quickly enter the tissues where they are transformed into tissue macrophages.

Macrophages are tissue phagocytes of long duration and acquire forms and functions depending on the tissue they populate. While neutrophils are short-lived (hours) and only reach inflamed tissues.

Activated macrophages are pro-inflammatory and secrete cytokines that activate the endothelium and neutrophils, causing the systemic manifestations of inflammation; but when the neutrophils end their function and die by apoptosis they are phagocytosed by the macrophages, becoming regulators that help the resolution of inflammation.

The hematopoietic organs in the fetus are the yolk sac, liver and spleen which produce monocytes that mainly populate the epidermis and CNS before the bone marrow takes over hematopoietic control.

NK cells are important in the defence against viruses and destroy tumour cells by ligand recognition with inhibitory and activating receptors. The balance between the activation of both types of receptors will determine whether the NK cell destroys the target cell and secretes cytokines or remains quiescent.

Inflammation is an immune defence response of the organism against aggressions, particularly infectious ones, and is characterized by 5 signs: redness, heat, pain, distention and functional impotence where oedema and leukocyte infiltration predominate.

The chronic inflammation occurs in days, weeks and months and involves innate response mechanisms with predominance of macrophages or eosinophils, but its perpetuation depends on the RIA where next to macrophages are Th1 lymphocytes to activate more macrophages and next to eosinophils Th2 that produces IL5 to increase eosinophils.

The effector mechanisms are dependent on the innate response, the acquired response or the amplification of the innate response by the acquired response. Adaptive effector mechanisms are mediated by antibodies and effector T lymphocytes. Antibodies neutralize viruses and toxins (IgM, IgG and IgAS) and exclude mucosal pathogens (IgAS). CTLs produce direct cytotoxicity of infected, mutated or tumour cells.

The amplification of innate mechanisms by acquired ones constitutes the majority of the effector mechanisms reinforcing the idea that IR is one and the same. Opsonophagocytosis is the process of facilitating phagocytosis by macrophages and neutrophils. It involves opsonins (antibodies and complement derivatives) that are recognized by specific receptors.

Apoptosis is a programmed, non-inflammatory and common mechanism of immune death employed by NKs and CTLs. During pregnancy, modifications occur in the mother's IS and uterine natural killer cells (NKu) appear. NKu are the most abundant cells in the placenta, endometrium and decidua and do not attack the trophoblast as they primarily recognize the MPP-G molecule.

There is a Th1/Th2 balance and, there is an increase in Treg cells during early pregnancy, an increase during the 2nd and 3rd trimester and then a decrease postpartum.

Mother and child

The mother protects, immunologically, the child from conception. She keeps it in a sterile environment preparing it for birth by transferring antibodies through the placenta, elaborated against previous maternal infections.

The mother-to-be should reactivate preventive vaccinations during pregnancy to increase the transfer of antibodies and the protection of her child. After birth, the mother provides other antibodies and cells through breast milk. She also provides non-pathogenic commensals to stimulate the mucosal immune system (SIM). These commensals are also provided by the vagina during natural childbirth, but not during cesarean section.

The protection transferred from the mother to the fetus and the newborn is exhausted in less than 6 months, during which time the newborn is developing its own defenses. However, this process leads to a natural and transitory deficiency of the IS, which explains the repeated infections of the child. Infections that should be left to run their course, if they are not serious.

During childhood there is a state of immunological immaturity, which generates susceptibility to infections that is compensated to some extent by maternal antibodies (IgG) that pass through the placenta during pregnancy and through breast milk (IgA).

Critical periods during life.

In the embryonic and foetal stage, the maternal IS must be able to protect the embryo and foetus against infections and, at the same time, to avoid the rejection of a new element with foreign components derived from the father, growing inside his organism. In the first year of life the newborn has a still immature IS, the protection depends to a great extent on the maternal antibodies that arrive through the placenta or breastfeeding in the first 6 months of life. In the infantile stage, as in the previous one, infections and contact with the external environment determine the maturation of the IS. At puberty the gradual involution of the thymus begins. Therefore, the full development of the IS in earlier stages is important to ensure good health in later stages. During pregnancy, changes in immune regulation occur that may promote the development of infections or modify the clinical course of various chronic conditions of the IS such as allergies and autoimmunities. During old age the process of immunosenescence causes a progressive erosion of immunosurveillance and an increased tendency to infections and tumours.

In the etiopathogenesis of diseases, knowing the essentials of Immunology in the healthy subject and the mechanisms involved in hypersensitivity disorders, will allow you to understand how diseases occur, what elements should be taken into account throughout the process, ie techniques that should be used for immunodiagnostics, how to cure them or at least alleviate them, which drugs affect the RI, which can be used and what prognosis to inform the patient.

During senescence, IS dysfunction occurs, characterized by decreased TCD4 and immunosurveillance (cancer), low-grade inflammation (chronic inflammation), loss of specificity (autoimmunity) and nutrition (susceptibility to infection).

Psychoneuroendocrineimmunology

Psychoneuroendocrineimmunology focuses on the bidirectional interactions between behavior (psyche), the *nervous system, the endocrine system and the immune system.* In the psyche the facts represent a minority and how one responds to them is what determines and that this integration overflows these systems interacting with the digestive, cardiovascular and reproductive, among others. These systems have in common that they are very complex with high levels of specialization and very efficient feedback; they have central and peripheral organs. The central organs of the central nervous system (CNS) are the brain with its hypothalamus; of the endocrine system the hypophysis or pituitary (adenohypophysis or anterior pituitary and neurohypophysis or posterior pituitary) and of the immune system, the bone marrow and thymus.

It is important to note that the endocrine hypophysis is within the CNS and that the hypothalamus produces a large amount of hormones, so it can also be considered endocrine. The peripheral organs of the nervous system are the vegetative or autonomic nervous system with its sympathetic and parasympathetic ganglia; endocrine are the adrenal glands, adrenal glands (ovary and testicle), thyroid and mammary glands among others; and immune are the secondary lymphoid organs (spleen, Waldeyer's ring, lymph nodes and appendix).

The CNS has ganglionic chains at the level of the sympathetic system and the immune system has ganglionic chains of lymph nodes.

The human CNS has the ability to learn and remember properties centered in the hippocampus. Learning primes the species with the legacy of previous generations. It has been postulated that adrenaline and cortisol secreted by the adrenal glands act on the am^gdala and then the hippocampus to induce memory. The RIA has arisen to learn and is characterized by the induction of immune memory, such as its ability to remember a first contact and subsequently respond to it in a more efficient way.

All three systems produce hormones, neuropeptides/neurotransmitters and cytokines. Hormones are any substance that is specifically secreted by a specialized cell and acts through a specialized receptor. All three systems express receptors for them at the cellular, tissue and organ level.

Hormone production occurs in the nervous, endocrine and immune systems. The CNS produces in the hypothalamus corticotropin releasing hormone (CRH); gonadotropin releasing hormone (GnRH); thyrotropin releasing hormone (TRH); growth hormone releasing hormone (GHRH); vasopressin and oxytocin which is stored in the neurohypophysis, dopamine, among others and also produces hormones at the peripheral nervous system level such as GR/epinephrine.

In response to hypothalamic hormones, the pituitary also produces several hormones at the central level: adenocorticotropin (ACTH); thyroid stimulating hormone (FSH); luteinizing hormone (LH); thyroid stimulating hormone (TSH), prolactin (PRL); releases stored antidiuretic hormone (ADH) or vasopressin and oxytocin, osteomyadipose growth hormone (GH) and at the peripheral level: thyroxine (T4) and triiodothyronine (T3) by the thyroid; glauco- and mineralo-corticoids, androgens and catecholamines (adrenaline and noradrenaline) and dehydroepiandrosterone (DHEA) by the adrenal cortex and angiotensin, epinephrine and norepinephrine by the adrenal medulla; estrogens and progesterone (ovary) and testosterone and androsterone (tesucles); milk production (breast) and leptin (adipocytes).

It produces hormones at central level (thymus) as: thymosin, thymulin, thymostimulin and thymopoietin that govern the differentiation and functionality of lymphocytes and erythropoietin at renal level that acts on the bone marrow for the production of erythrocytes and at peripheral level mast cells produce histamine and serotonin and these and eosinophils produce prostaglandins and leukotrienes. Thymopoietin is also involved in the neuromuscular transmission interacting with the CNS and thymulin mainly increases the activity of Treg.

The CNS establishes communication with secondary lymphoid organs such as lymph nodes through the vegetative system via the sympathetic and parasympathetic system nerves activating or inhibiting multiple functions in various organs. The sympathetic system inhibits the action of adrenaline and noradrenaline on the SI. The vagus efferent produces acetylcholine (main neurotransmitter) which acts by inhibiting existing receptors on IS cells such as macrophages. The hypothalamus produces CRH which acts on the adenohypophysis to produce ACTH which in turn activates the adrenal gland to produce cortisol, stress hormone, catecholamines and dehydroepiandrosterone (DHEA) which acts on gonads to produce estrogen or testosterone. Cortisol and adrenaline are involved in the induction of memory by the CNS. Cortisol is immunosuppressive on lymphocytes, macrophages and inflammation and inhibits the pituitary and hypothalamus, as well as interfering with fertility. Estrogens inhibit mammary secretion and prolactin inhibits ovulation. Glucagon and insulin produced by the pancreas regulate blood sugar levels and somatostatin, also produced by the pancreas, inhibits the pituitary.

The IS is programmed to contract following contact with the anUgen, possesses Treg that inhibit the stimulation of different RI patterns and induces cytokine-mediated cross-regulation.

Neurons and endocrine gland cells, like all nucleated cells, express MPP-I. These molecules are essential in immune defences as they are involved in the presentation of peptides to TCD8 and are used by neurons in interneuronal communication and by neurons with the IS and function to ensure protection and return to homeostasis.

The CNS through the basic emotions (anger, fear, disgust, pleasure, sadness, surprise and contempt) defends itself with generally transient reactions (acute stress) to return to homeostasis. The IS defends itself through the innate response and if this is not able to eliminate the danger it triggers the RIA mechanisms. The IS is also programmed to repair the damage and return to homeostasis.

Patterns of defense

The patterns of defense where several systems interact are the *production of fever, hormone production, cytokines at the cellular level and nitric oxide.*

In the face of infection, the production of proinflammatory cytokines is stimulated by resident cells such as macrophages and mast cells at the site of infection. TNF and IL1 are hormone-acting cytokines that travel to the hypothalamus via the vagus nerve (afferent pathway) to induce fever and attempt to limit the inflammatory response via the efferent sympathetic pathway. Fever acts at the level of the inflamed site by increasing the chemotaxis of neutrophils and T lymphocytes; in the nervous system, in the brain, it produces drowsiness and anorexia to decrease metabolism and energy consumption; in the muscles by increasing protein catabolism and the availability of amino acids and in the intestine it stimulates the synthesis of acute phase proteins (haptoglobulin, fibrinogen, CRP, amyloid A, among others); the endocrine system increases the production of insulin, glucagon, growth hormone, TSH and vasopressin; the bone marrow (neutrophilia, anemia and decreases serum iron removed by lactoferrin; repair increases fibroblasts to form collagen; B cells proliferation and production of antibodies, Th (activation and production of IL2) and cytotoxic T cells; IFN type I production and oxidative activity of phagocytes. Consequently, increased fever has antiviral and antibacterial actions. It should be remembered that in addition to infections, fever can be induced by: non-infectious inflammation including autoimmunity; tissue necrosis (post-infarction); metallopoxemia (gout and porphyria) and tumors (solid and hematologic);

Mast cells produce histamine and serotonin and these and eosinophils produce prostaglandins and leukotrienes. Activated lymphocytes produce hormones and neurotransmitters. These include: gonadotrophin, ACTH, TSH, prolactin, growth hormone, corticosteroids, catecholamines, acetylcholine, endorphins and enkephalins. TNF induces ACTH secretion by leukocytes. Neuropeptides also activate mast cells. IL7 which triggers T and B growth is produced by central immune organs and various cells of the innate response, as well as hepatocytes and neurons;

As part of the IS, the complement system is involved in energy metabolism in peripheral nerves and signal transduction in the CNS;

Metric oxide is a neurotransmitter constitutively produced by neurons. It is also constitutively produced by vascular endothelium to maintain vascular tone. Metric oxide is also an effector of phagocyte IR induced by the action of metric oxide synthase on arginine;

Evidence for psychoneuroendocrine-immune interactions
Among the most significant are *breastfeeding; the effect of sex hormones during gestation and climacteric; responses to infection, ischemia or other insult; and, stress as an immunosuppressant.*
Milk secretion is inhibited by dopamine produced by the hypothalamus. Initially it is necessary to produce GHRH by the hypothalamus to induce PRL secretion by the adenohypophysis. PRL stimulates the mammary alveoli which together with oxytocin produced by the hypothalamus and stored in the neurohypophysis contracts the alveolar muscles to produce milk. Other prolactin stimulating factors are: GnRH, TRH, estrogen and vasoactive intestinal polypeptide. If the mother is not psychically prepared to want to produce milk for her baby or thinks that breastfeeding will alter her beauty, neither PRL nor milk is produced. The suckling performed by the baby stimulates the hypothalamic sensory receptors so that more PRL is produced.
During gestation hormonal changes occur as one of the factors that tend to avoid the rejection of the semiallogeneic fetus. Firstly, the chorionic gonadotrophin increases in the first trimester and later, estrogens and progesterone increase progressively in the 2nd and 3rd trimester to fall drastically at the end of pregnancy. In the 3rd age comes the climacteric period in women where there is a great decrease in the production of estrogens;
When an infection occurs, macrophages and mast cells produce an acute phase response including the cytokines TNF, IL1, IL6 which travel along the afferent vagus nerve to the CNS. The CNS receives the information, integrates it and coordinates the response. Initially, the hypothalamus increases the temperature producing fever. At the same time, it produces CRH which, acting on the adenohypophysis, produces ACTH. This activates the adrenal to produce cortisol, adrenaline and noradrenaline. Additionally, the hypothalamus sends the neurotransmitter, acetylcholine, through the vagus efferent for which there are receptors at the level of the cells of the innate immune system. Subsequently, the sympathetic peripheral system inhibits the actions of adrenaline and noradrenaline. Thus, cortisol, the interaction of acetylcholine

with its receptor and the blockade of adrenaline and noradrenaline are aimed at limiting inflammation. In the particular case of a hand burn, the sensory nerve endings send a painful stimulus to the CNS which immediately responds with an automatic motor nerve action to withdraw the hand. Finally, macrophages are in charge of repairing the damaged tissue to return it to homeostasis;

Stress has multiple causes that can be grouped into *biogenic* (extreme temperature, intense exercise, poor digestion, pain from an injury, memory of an unpleasant situation) and *biopsychosocial* (workload, couple arguments, fear of speaking in public, intense noise or light) particularly those associated with the challenging society and the comforts in which we live. These can be acute or chronic and are fundamentally mediated by the production of cortisol which has been called the stress hormone.

Acute stress lasts for minutes or hours, aims to redistribute leukocytes to the site of aggression and increases innate and acquired primary and secondary responses being consequently immunopotentiating. Consequently, they affect the affective-emotional behavior and the degree of alertness of the organism with beneficial actions. In acute stress the stressors were related to the physical survival of the species such as: the need to obtain food; to shelter; to defend itself and to procreate. This adapts the organism to respond quickly to challenges so that we strike back or have a strategic retreat. This response of "attack or flight" happens at the level of the neurovegetative system, that is to say, it is not conscious, on the contrary, it is automatic. We do not decide but it is the organism that recognizes the need to respond and does it automatically, similar to when we drive or increase the heart rate, temperature and sweating when we run.

Chronic stress lasts for weeks or years, decreases innate (NK, phagocytes) and acquired responses, affects the cardiovascular and renal systems, produces physical exhaustion, weight loss, stomach and digestive disorders, and decreases sensory and intellectual responses, thus being immunosuppressive. Our society does not allow us to fight physically or escape when we face stressors; but neither does it eliminate them, on the contrary, it increases them. Today stressors are more associated with professional and social success and with satisfying one's own and others' social expectations. This leads us to be on constant alert, ready for action that we often do not execute and we begin to feel its effects. Thus, the Kmbic system (emotional responses) is chronically activated with the secretion of ACTH and endorphins, producing more cortisol and not adrenaline, which leads to harmful effects: effects on the cardiovascular and renal system (hyperglycemia, acidosis, dehydration, electrolyte anomaKas, physical exhaustion and weight loss); hardening of the arteries due to increased circulating cholesterol; digestive disorders; effects on body temperature; increased sensitivity with headaches and back pain; increased ulcerations; rebound of allergic reactions; decreased sensory and intellectual responses; sexual problems; increased blood circulation disorders; increased processes of lipolysis, glycogenesis and cytogenesis and changes in the pattern of functioning of immune markers such as T lymphocytes, NK cells, immunoglobulins, erythrosedimentation and rheumatoid factor, antibodies to Epstein-Barr virus and tuberculin reaction.

Stress stimulates the central nervous and neurovegetative systems to produce CRH and TRH by the hypothalamus. These activate the adenohypophysis of the endocrine system producing ACTH and TSH. These activate the adrenal glands producing catecholamines (adrenaline and noradrenaline) and cortisol and the thyroid (producing thyroid hormones), respectively.

The dynamics of these actions can be seen in the mobilization of energy, energy support systems, mobilization of auxiliary resources and defensive reactions.

For energy mobilization, *adrenaline* acts at the systemic level and *noradrenaline* at the local level, at the nerve endings of the neurovegetative system, in the adrenal medulla and in the ascending and descending brainstem. These are powerful stimulants that speed up reflexes, increase heart rate and blood pressure, raise blood sugar concentration and accelerate metabolism. Thyroid hormones secreted by the thyroid gland into the bloodstream further increase metabolism and increase the amount of energy that can be consumed. They release hepatic cholesterol into the bloodstream, increasing energy and aiding muscle function;

The energy support system is seen in the suppression of digestive function by diverting blood from the stomach to the lungs and muscles and inducing dryness of the mouth. Diverting blood from the skin to the lungs and muscles with pallor characteristic of states of intense stress and increased sweating, to help overheated muscles cool down and regulate. Increased oxygenation of the blood by the dilated lungs with increased breathing rate;

In the mobilization of auxiliary resources, endorphins are released by the neurohypophysis which act as natural painkillers and reduce sensitivity to injuries such as bruises and wounds. Cortisol is released which prevents allergic reactions that can interfere with breathing. It sharpens the senses and increases mental performance. The production of sex hormones is decreased, which prevents the diversion of energy to these functions.

For defensive reactions, the blood vessels are constricted and the blood is thickened to slow down the flow of blood so that it coagulates more quickly in case of injury.

Thus, chronic stress is somatized by signs and symptoms of other illnesses such as when a loved one dies, often one becomes ill with influenza. In long-term couples the death of the spouse depresses the other and the death usually comes before the age of 2 years.

When we are subjected to sustained tension at work due to disagreements with colleagues or the boss, skin diseases and infections usually appear;

When there are sustained socio-economic stresses such as job loss, lack of money, break-ups and marital problems we generally get sick; and when immunosuppressive drugs are taken, infections increase.

There are hormones associated with happiness such as dopamine for pleasure and motivation and serotonin for mood; endorphins (joy and well-being) and adrenaline. One way to stimulate them is by activating vital activity, sexuality.

As we saw before, the nervous, endocrine and immune systems are very complex and specialized; with central and peripheral organs, capable of learning and memory; they function through mediators, particularly hormones and their receptors; highly regulated; all nucleated cells, including neurons, express MPP-I.

Hormones are an important example of the interactions of these systems acting in chains where one activates another and produces actions that feed back into the system.

SI Laboratory Tests

This defense system protects us from infections from both outside and inside the body. All diseases suffered by the body, from the most common (cold, flu, allergies,...) to serious diseases, have a response based on the state of the IS. Immunological tests can be grouped into those that evaluate innate or acquired responses and those that evaluate cells, their function and the molecules produced.

The cellular tests that evaluate the innate response are: leukogram with differential; peripheral laminin; erythrocyte sedimentation and immunophenotyping.

Innate functional tests include: phagocytosis in all its steps; NK activity and antibody amplified (ADCC, basophilic degranulation and passive cutaneous anaphylaxis).

The innate tests where the molecules produced are evaluated are: PCR, complement, cytokines and natural and universal antibodies.

The cellular tests acquired are: the lymphocyte count in the leukogram with differential and peripheral lamina and immunophenotyping.

Acquired functional tests include: proliferation against mitogens and anrigens of T and B lymphocytes; cytotoxic activity of TCD8; lymphocytotoxicity; delayed hypersensitivity and immediate hypersensitivity. The acquired tests where the molecules produced are evaluated are: protein electrophoresis and the quantification of cytokines and immunoglobulins. Other tests are the quantification of cytokines, cell signaling proteins, soluble proteins and immunoglobulins by multiparametric immunoassay by flow cytometry according to the CBA Kits method.

Polyclonal and monoclonal antibodies are frequently used to identify and quantify T and B lymphocyte populations, subpopulations, cell development and function.

The main immunological methods to determine the anUgen-antibody interaction are based on particle agglutination, immunocomplex precipitation and enzyme labeling using either fluorochromes or radioisotopes.

Bibliography

Abul K Abbas, Andrew H Lichtman, Shiv Pillai. Inmunolog^a celular y molecular Octava edicion. Spain Elsevier 2015

Quantification of cytokines, cell signaling proteins, soluble proteins and immunoglobulins by multiparametric flow cytometric immunoassay. Method cba. www.ibsgranada.es

Kindt TJ, Goldsby RA and Osborne BA. Kuby's Immunology^a Sixth edition McGRAW-HILL Interamericana Editores, S.A. de C.V. 2007

Palomo GI, Ferreira VA, Sepulveda CC, Rosemblatt SM, Vergara CU. Fundamentals of Basic and Clinical Immunology. Talca Chile, 2009

Perez Martm O G, Vega Garrta Irma G. La Inmunolog^a en el humano sano para estudiantes de Ciencias Medicas. Havana, Medical Sciences 2017: 6-56.

Chapter, 2
Eosinophilic esophagitis

Dr. Cristian Ponce Alvarez and Dr. Gabriela Jardines Arciniega

Introduction

Eosinophilic esophagitis (EoE) is a chronic inflammatory disease of the esophagus, characterized by clinical symptoms of esophageal dysfunction, and histologically due to inflammation of the esophagus, where eosinophils usually dominate, there are more than 15 eosinophils per high magnification field (EOS / CGA). Currently, it is considered to be mainly caused by non-IgE-mediated food allergy, but not limited to food amphigens. Being a chronic disease from the point of view of incidence and prevalence, the initial characterization of EoE as a clinical pathological syndrome of its own, distinct from eosinophilic gastroenteritis, was made in the early 1990s by two independent research teams in the United States and Switzerland. EoE is no longer a rare disease and affects at least 1 in 1000-2000 European and North American residents aged 5 and 6 years, the recent incidence for children and adults reported from Spain (about 100 cases per 100,000 inhabitants). The results are as mentioned above, EoE currently means that it is the second leading cause of chronic esophagitis, after gastroesophageal reflux disease (GERD) and the leading cause of dysphagia and indigestion in children and young people. The reason is unknown because foods consumed by humans since the NeoKthic; such as milk, wheat, eggs and beans, have started to cause this disease in the last 25 years, although it is suspected that multiple factors such as modern lifestyle (improved hygienic conditions, changes in food types, consumption, genetic manipulation and contamination from chemical additives and animal husbandry with hormones and antibiotics, as well as secondary changes in the human intestinal microbiota may be involved in the genesis of the disease.

Pathophysiological basis of esophagitis The pathophysiological mechanism of EoE some authors agree that it is an inflammatory process of immunological cause, determined by a possible hypersensitivity to certain dietary ingredients or airborne allergens. This theory is supported by the following facts: patients with personal and family medical history with asthma, allergic rhinitis, atopic dermatitis, drug and food allergy, blood eosinophilia or increased serum IgE values. Positive skin allergy tests and radioabsorbance allergy tests (RAST) have also been reported. In addition, remission of histological lesions has been reported in subjects following elemental diets lacking antigenic capacity. It seems obvious that eosinophils play an important role in the development of

EoE-related dysphagia, especially when these patients respond satisfactorily to the use of antieosinophilic therapy. More than ten years ago, it was established that in the presence of GERD the number of esophageal T lymphocytes increases, recently it has been confirmed that in EoE the number of these cells also significantly increased the number of CD3+ cells and CD4+ and CD8+ subsets in pediatric and adult cases with EoE with respect to healthy controls. Mast cells are also involved in the immunoallergic reaction and are increased in the esophageal epithelium in EoE. In the confocal microscopy study in food allergy, mast cells were observed in the afferent nerve fiber, causing membrane potential instability and consequently causing muscle contraction. This causes movement disorders following the release of granules in the digestive system in these patients by activation of receptors for high affinity IgE-containing particles (FC£RI) or non-immunologic response. Few studies have aimed to identify B lymphocytes in the esophageal mucosa, although fewer T lymphocytes seem to be related. However, plasma cells that secrete large amounts of IgE have been identified in the esophageal epithelium, which does not express CD19 or CD20 markers of the B lymphocytes from which they originate, although primary eosinophil infiltration of the esophagus may be due to a TH2 cell-type immune response, the available data conclude that B cell- and IgE-dependent humoral immunity play an important role in the initiation or maintenance of the esophageal eosinophilic infiltrate. The signal transduction process of eosinophil recruitment is involved in gastrointestinal diseases, these cells appear to respond to biological stimuli generally. Thus, activation of the local inflammatory response determines the expression of interleukin on vascular endothelial cell adhesion. (IL)-1в and tumor necrosis factor alpha (TNFa), responsible for adhesion and extravasation of eosinophils. Most of the research on eosinophil recruitment to tissues is done in the lungs. In chronic allergic reactions, IL-5 plays an indispensable role, which is an important factor in the proliferation, differentiation, survival and activation of eosinophils, T-helper lymphocytes and mast cells. IL-5 has been clearly involved in the pathophysiology and fiber remodeling of allergic asthma that occurs in chronic bronchial and cutaneous inflammation. By studying this cytokine in EoE he has developed a transgenic mouse overexpressing IL-5, which has an increase of circulating eosinophils in the blood and a large accumulation of eosinophils in the esophageal lamina propria. Conversely, mice lacking this cytokine did not develop esophageal eosinophilia when exposed to gas-sensitive allergens via the inhalation route. These findings clearly indicate that a TH2-like immune response is involved in the pathogenesis of EoE. A new study analyzed the gene expression of different cytokines in the esophageal epithelium of children with EoE compared to "healthy" controls, and also defined the average overexpression of IL-5 in children with EoE. IL-3 and GM-CSF are also directly involved, proliferate and accumulate with IL-5, the eosinophil response to allergens. Additionally, tissue eosinophils and activated eosinophils can produce these cytokines, especially GM-CSF, so there may be an autocrine process that is at least partially responsible for the survival and accumulation of eosinophils in tissue. So far, no studies have confirmed the gene expression of this gene. These cytokines are in EoE, but we have some experience in animal models, which may support this fact. Chemokines are a subfamily of chemokines (contains 3 molecules called eosinophil-activating chemokines 1, 2 and 3), through the chemokine receptor (CCR)-3 which is mainly found on these white blood cells, can act as a powerful and specific chemoattractant for eosinophils. Eotaxin-1 (CCL11) is the most studied chemokine in the digestive tract, it is widely expressed in the digestive tract and its mRNA can be obtained from monocytes residing in the lamina propria of rat small intestine, which is the area where most eosinophils live in the digestive tract under normal conditions. Studies in mice lacking eotaxin-1 have shown that they have fewer eosinophils in all parts of the gastrointestinal tract, because the lack of eotaxin prevents the recruitment of eosinophils to the gastrointestinal tract, thereby increasing the amount of eosinophils in the circulation. Thus, even in the presence of elevated levels of IL-5, eosinophil eotaxin is essential for eosinophil recruitment to the gastrointestinal tract, but does not modify their presence in the bone marrow or peripheral blood. This indicates that the effect of eosinophil eotaxin-1 is tissue specific and its expression does not affect the production of eosinophils in bone marrow or the circulating value of these white blood cells. Elevated eotaxin-1 is associated with various inflammatory diseases of the human respiratory tract and is related to the clinical severity of the process. Although eosinophil eotaxin-1 may be related to the pathophysiology of human EoE, despite the presence of large numbers of intraepithelial eosinophils, no increase in serum eosinophil eotaxin expression was observed in these patients. In the USA, recent research has focused on eotaxin-3 (CCL26) may play the major role in the process of studying the pathophysiology of EoE, it was found that, compared to healthy individuals, the eotaxin-3 gene is induced with higher intensity in EoE patients, however, other results from a group of children with EoE show overexpression compared to control, eotaxin-1 and RANTES expression appears to be suppressed. RANTES (regulated upon activation, normal T-cells expressedand secreted chemokine) is another chemokine involved in the inflammatory process and compared to mouse EoE, is slightly upregulated in epithelial cells, data that humans cannot confirm. RANTES and eotaxin, both produced by inflammatory cells, cannot be detected in esophageal epithelial cells, indicating that eosinophils themselves, and certainly RANTES, are not sufficient to recruit and infiltrate the esophagus. Therefore, IL-5 produced by T lymphocytes may be other factors necessary for eosinophil infiltration, with the exception of eotaxin and RANTES. These results are limited by the fact that they are obtained by analyzing cell population and cytokine expression in the esophageal epithelium, and cannot predict the behavior of inflammatory infiltration of lower layers such as the submucosa in areas of organs with higher cell density that are normally immune. The TH2 type reaction is mainly mediated. Through CD4+ helper T lymphocytes, but some previous results have confirmed that EoE inflammatory infiltration is mainly CD8+, traditionally considered TH1 cytokine-secreting lymphocytes such as interferon gamma (IFN) and TNF are clear markers. Straumann et al found that TNF values were elevated in esophageal biopsies from 8 adult patients with EoE, and Gupta et al reported increased IFN gene expression in a series of children with this disease, therefore, we should consider the possibility that the TH1-mediated inflammatory cascade may also play a role in the pathogenesis of EoE.

On the other hand, for several reasons, EoE is not necessarily a local disease limited to the organ; for one thing, the increased number of eosinophils in the blood of many patients may respond to bone marrow stimulation. Secondly, many patients showing signs of inflammation in other organs (such as bronchial asthma, rhinoconjunctivitis or atopic dermatitis) may mean that the esophageal events are part of a systemic allergic disease. For these reasons, many authors caution that EoE may not be an independent pathologic process, but only a clinical expression in the general allergic constitution of these patients.

Epidemiolog^a

EoE is clearly an emerging entity. To date, about 140 articles have documented different cases of eosinophilic esophagitis in children and adult patients, among them, 75% have been published in the last 5 years. On the one hand, this fact can be explained by the increased incidence and prevalence of this disease, which may coincide with the common cause of the increase of allergic diseases in recent decades, related to atopic reaction, residents of industrialized countries; On the other hand, with regard to the knowledge of the existence of this disease among physicians, the disease began to be considered in the differential diagnosis of dysphagia and esophageal stricture, of course, pathologists also connote this disease, this is the key to the process of diagnosis of EoE. Straumann's estimates from his Swiss adult case series collected an incidence rate of 57-59 years over 16 years, 1,438 cases per 100,000 population. In recent years, newly diagnosed cases have increased and the prevalence rate is 23 cases per 100,000 population. Noel et al, estimated that children in EoE vwan epidemiology in an area of Ohio (United States): from their records, they estimated an incidence of 10 children per 100,000 population each year at the end of 2003, and found an incidence of 43 cases per 100,000 population, these data indicate that EoE vwan in an area of Ohio (United States): from their records, they estimated an incidence of 10 children per 100,000 population each year at the end of 2003, and found an incidence of 43 cases per 100,000 population.These data indicate that the incidence of EoE in industrialized countries is at least as high as other recognized entities with gastrointestinal inflammation, such as Crohn's disease (in the United States, the incidence varies from 3.6 to 8.8 cases per 100,000 inhabitants per year) and proposed that the incidence of EoE in industrialized countries is at least as high as other recognized entities with gastrointestinal inflammation, such as Crohn's disease.000 inhabitants per year) and proposed that although EoE has not been considered an extremely rare disease, based on manifestations in adulthood, the actual frequency of occurrence is much higher than a priori expectations and may exceed the frequency of other chronic inflammatory diseases of the digestive tract, Moreover, considering the gradual increase in the incidence of EoE, it is foreseeable that in the coming years it will continue to increase despite the lack of knowledge to obtain general information about this entity among physicians, it remains an underdiagnosed entity, and we only focus on the "tip of the iceberg". In both children and adults, EoE affects mainly males according to a review of a large number of cases in childhood, more than 65% of all diagnosed disease in the adult form, and is most often described in subjects between the third and fifth decade of life.

Clinical Aspects

The natural history of EoE has not yet been defined, however, the long duration of symptoms before diagnosis and the length of time between the absence of symptoms indicate that adult EoE is both a chronic disease and an insensitive disease.

In an extensive review of different publications involving 200 patients, Fox compiled different clinical symptoms related to this entity and observed significant differences in clinical manifestations between children and adults (Table I), other aspects also noted at this point in more recent studies. Although there is no explanation for the reasons for these differences, it is speculated that they are closely related to the timing of the disease or the duration of exposure of the esophagus to eosinophil infiltration, food bolus impaction in the esophagus is the most common clinical manifestation leading to diagnosis in adult patients and occurs in more than 20% of cases of childhood disease. Recent reviews in the medical literature estimate that food impaction in the esophagus occurs in 56% to 88% of adults affected by eosinophilic esophagitis. Esophageal calcifications are small or even normal; many involve persistent effects that require immediate endoscopic resolution, although they may be self-limiting and patients usually adapt to these episodes. Clinical symptoms (chronic dysphagia, dysphagia of variable duration with acute on-off phenomenon, food impaction in the esophagus) necessarily involve esophageal smooth muscle contraction, reminiscent of bronchial smooth muscle contraction. In this regard, studies in mice have shown that eosinophilic inflammation of the respiratory tract is closely related to esophageal inflammation. There is evidence that eosinophilic infiltration of the digestive system is associated with weight loss and gastric dysmotility. These are from animal models and human observations.

TABLE I_ **Symptoms associated with eosinofflc esophagitis**

Adults
   Dysphagia
   Food impact
   Vomiting, ejTiesis
   DDI or thoracic
Children
   Dysphagia
   Food impact
   Vomiting, emesis, regurgitation
   Chest pain
   Nnnseas
   Piro sis
   H ipe rя 11 i vaciotn
   Coinpcirtaniictyl aliinentary avrersive. hypocrecijniento
   Doi or abdominal epi^astrico
   S into mas respiratory: cough, stridor^ sinusitis* obstiuccicn neli mon i a

Ktodi fi cadc < ic Fox et ala.

Diagnostic

Endoscopy

On endoscopic findings, the change in the caliber of the esophageal cavity has been described as regular concentric stricture or presence of segmental rings at the same time, which prevents the observation of the distal cavity and the development of endoscopy, without the mucosa associated with lesions, which are cause of food impaction. Other more subtle findings are longitudinal linear grooves and white punctate or papular exudate, indicating the presence of mucus deposits or microabscesses composed of eosinophils. Patients with EoE showed very diverse changes in the pattern of the esophageal mucosa, the two most commonly observed changes on endoscopy are: irregular appearance of the mucosa, more or less elevated external papules and longitudinal linear grooves that extend along the organ and are deposited in the esophageal folds. When collapsed, this type of groove, also known as esophageal "corrugation", is up to 97% of the cases described in the Australian series. Characteristic esophageal tears have also been described after endoscopic dilatation. Stenosis is rarely described in children. Endoscopy of other patients was normal. Barium radiology studies may occasionally show the presence of stricture or cleft. Ring patterns are usually normal, some authors even suggest that dye reactive dye methods with a contrast medium nebulizer or chromoendoscopy may reveal these lesions, but this is not very obvious.

Histology

In many cases there is no endoscopic result. The characteristics of the mucosa of the organ make the diagnostic criterion of EoE. There is a dense infiltration of the esophageal mucosa, each field of view consists of more than 20 eosinophils, high magnification (CGA) (400) has been established as the standard for differential histopathology. However, in a few control individuals, due to the presence of CGA, the number of eosinophils infiltrating the esophageal epithelium did not exceed 2-3 per field, which may be part of the normal histology of the distal third of the organ. GERD is the most common cause of esophageal eosinophils, the number of eosinophils is also very low and the cell density of each EGC does not exceed 7-10 eosinophils per field. All described lesions respond to the same pattern of histopathological lesions, which are characterized by epithelial edema, increased intercellular spaces, increased epithelial cells, and at the expense of hyperproliferative changes, infiltration of inflammatory cells and varying degrees of expression.

Esophageal manometry

There are few cases to study esophageal motor function and the results are not uniform, since different movement disorders have been defined in EoE, of which the most frequent are non-specific.

Landres describes the case diagnosed as patient Eosinophilic gastroenteritis with esophageal infection, he presented a movement disorder, which corresponds to a vigorous achalasia, so he underwent an extramucosal myotomy according to the technique described by Heller. The biopsy of the esophageal muscle layer showed hypertrophy, in addition to a massive infiltration of eosinophils, esophageal manifestations of the disease are secondary to the disease. Endoscopic ultrasonography of eosinophilic esophagitis showed thickening of the esophageal mucosa and submucosa, as well as of the muscle layer, although the latter observation may also signify increased muscle tone. Eosinophil protein has also been detected by specific staining in extracellular tissues, patients with gastrointestinal eosinophilic disease and in specimens from patients with EoE. In particular, the major basic protein (MBP) is the most abundant toxin contained in the cytoplasmic granules of eosinophils, and in addition to being a potent agonist, it is also directly related to those observed in eosinophilic diseases and the cytotoxicity is directly related. The latter, which binds to the M2 muscarinic acetylcholine receptor, directs the contractile function of the smooth muscle of the gastrointestinal tract, which constitutes two-thirds of the distal esophagus. Direct stimulation of MBP can directly increase smooth muscle responsiveness and excessive contractility, which can be detected by manometric studies. Histological studies on food allergy by confocal microscopy showed that mast cells are located near afferent nerve fibers and their histamine degranulation can change the stability of neuronal membranes. Mast cell granules also contain leukotriene C4, which is a direct stimulus of smooth muscle contraction. In a detailed review of the medical literature, we found 84 cases of esophageal eosinophilic infiltration, in which manometric recordings were used to study organ motor function (Table II). This group included 38 children, and the other 2 cases were diagnosed as esophageal infiltrative eosinophilic gastroenteritis. For these reasons, only a total of 46 adult patients whose esophageal motor function was assessed by manometry have been reported in the medical literature. Of the 84 patients with eosinorilic esophageal infiltration described, 55 have detected different types of manometric disorders (65.5% of the overall series), representing all types of movement disorders, mostly spastic or excessive contractility. Thus, the medical literature describes dyskinesias in EoE, which meet the criteria of severe portal achalasia, diffuse esophageal spasm, "nutcracker" esophagus or presence of high amplitude peristaltic waves 98100. A review of the medical literature also showed that normal esophageal movements were observed in most patients.

Treatment

There is little evidence to show what is the best treatment for patients with EoE. The paucity of reported cases and the fact of chronic disease mean that the current treatment methods used in these patients are still controversial and the need for maintenance treatment is unknown. On the other hand, it is unclear whether patients with asymptomatic esophageal eosinophilia should be treated during the crisis and whether this will affect the medium or long-term course of the disease. The only published study analyzing the long-term clinical course of EoE-related symptoms shows that eosinophil infiltration persists in all symptomatic patients, it is said that without treatment, fibrosis of the organ wall is secondary to inflammation, which will lead to irreversible impairment of the organ's motor function. For this reason, the authors of the study recommend esophageal dilation as the therapy of choice, other authors do not. Below, we summarize the different treatment options tested in EoE.

Dietetic treatment

Dietary restrictions and basic diet has been shown to be effective in many pediatric age cases, but its high cost and difficult compliance make it a less suitable treatment option, especially if we consider it a chronic disease. In the case of adult patients, these difficulties are even more prominent. The dietary treatment is the long-term avoidance of only those foods that have been shown to cause the disease, after their individual reintroduction.

Pharmacological treatment

For ameliorating clinical symptoms and reversing histologic lesions, systemic corticosteroids have been shown to be effective, but have side effects that limit their use. Recently, topical corticosteroids have been tried, especially fluticasone propionate, which are equivalent in efficacy to systemic corticosteroids, but lack many side effects and are well tolerated by patients. In particular, patients who have received clinical, endoscopic and histological data that have responded to PPIs constitute the subphenotype of patients with EoE. In contrast to all previous clinical guidelines, response to PPIs excludes the presence of EoE. Several recent studies have shown that the molecular expression of EoE patients are similar. It has also been confirmed that PPIs can play the same role, at the molecular level, in desinflammation as topical swallowed corticosteroids. Considering that EoE symptoms usually recur 3 to 6 months after discontinuation of drug treatment, two recent prospective series of patients have shown that patients responding to corticosteroids or elimination diet also respond to treatment with PPIs, and vice versa. Therefore, the choice of an initial treatment does not preclude the patient from being transferred to another anti-inflammatory treatment during the course of the disease. For other possible treatment methods of application, such as mast cell membrane stabilizing drugs or leukotriene inhibitors, there is insufficient experience.

Although there are currently no sperm preparations for the treatment of EoE, several randomized trials using topical corticosteroids in children and adults have been conducted, summarizing several systematic reviews and meta-analyses. These studies have confirmed that these drugs have a high efficacy in inducing histological remission of EoE. However, due to the inclusion criteria, the drugs used (fluticasone or budesonide), the daily dose, the duration of treatment (2 to 12 weeks) and the difference in application methods, the comparative interpretation of the results is complicated. Medications (dry powder inhalers, variable viscosity suspensions, or effervescent dispersible oral dispersible tablets), and the criteria defining histologic relief (<1 to <20 EOS/CGA). However, it seems clear that the drug delivery system along the esophagus is essential to obtain adequate and continuous mucosal coverage of the organs, avoiding the deposition of corticosteroids in other tissues.

Dosis recomendadas para la inducción y el mantenimiento de la enfermedad con IBP y corticoides tópicos deglutidos.

	Inducta cin		Marten I mi ento	
	N1 us	Adults	Children	Adults
Proton pump inhibitors (PPIs)	1-2 mg/kg/din* 1-2 mg/kg/din* 1-2 mg/kg/din* 1-2 mg/kg/din	Omeprazole 20--40 orc each t 2li	1 mg/kg/ dia20-40	Omeprazole mg every 24ti
Topical curtico ides ofgl irtildos				
Fl LIticusomi	1600-1 760	mcg/dfa* mcg/dfa	SBO-1 760 mcgZdia*.	
B ml that iild a	1-2 m<j/d la*	2-4 riHj'dla*	Similar to ізогонот	

Divided into two daily intakes.¹
Multiple studies have demonstrated a substantial loss of response with oral viscous budescjnide СЗО-ТОЧЙ3 when the dose that led to remission during induction is reduced. ⁴⁻⁴⁷

Endoscopic treatments

Patients with EoE are susceptible to the influence of food and the development of esophageal strictures. In this regard, endoscopy or esophageal dilation are treatment options to be considered. Because of their different meanings, we will discuss them separately: - Esophageal impaction is the most common manifestation leading to the diagnosis of EoE and requires urgent endoscopic resolution. In your clinical evaluation, you should look for the presence of past or recurrent effects and a personal history of allergies. In addition, endoscopy allows you to evaluate for the presence of esophageal strictures or esophageal rings and mucosal appearance of the organ. In the presence of mucosal changes suspicious for EoE, biopsies for diagnostic purposes should be considered during the same endoscopic procedure or on a deferred basis.

- Endoscopic dilatations are the common treatment for rigid or fibrous esophageal strictures resulting from the healing of long-lasting inflammatory processes, affecting the lining of the digestive tract and can expand the lumen of the organ by tearing the fibrous structures of its wall. With this in mind, several authors have resorted to hydropneumatic dilatation of esophageal mucosal strictures by its eosinophilic infiltration, undoubtedly providing symptomatic relief in an immediate manner, so that some authors have suggested it as the treatment of choice for EoE even though it does not act on the inflammatory substrate of the underlying EoE. Chest pain has been reported as a complication of this technique in EoE. Hospitalization and intravenous analgesia and bleeding from unusual tears, hematomas, and perforations have been requested. Therefore, steroid therapy should be considered when EoE is suspected in patients with esophageal dysphagia and strictures for topical use, and endoscopic expansion should not be performed until eosinophil infiltration is ruled out.

Experience reported so far on the evaluation of the effects of different EoE treatments has used the normalization of morphological changes observed in samples of esophageal mucosa as a criterion of response to treatment, including the disappearance of dense eosinophilic infiltration. Studies to evaluate the degree of symptom relief have not yet established objective or quantifiable criteria for clinical improvement. In this sense, we currently lack tools to evaluate the response to treatment, which cannot verify the therapeutic effects of different immunomorphologies, symptoms and functions of this disease. Moreover, since there are no controlled studies comparing different treatment modalities in terms of efficacy or safety, although it seems logical to make topical steroid therapy the first choice for its usefulness, it is difficult to establish an adequate course of action, being assessed by different studies and its safety in children and adults.

Forecast

Knowledge about the natural history of EoE is limited and not fully defined in many respects. The available data do not indicate that EoE affects life expectancy or is associated with cancer, but it is of concern that chronic uncontrolled inflammation may cause irreversible structural damage to the esophagus, leading to fibrosis, stricture, and changes in esophageal function. Increased time of untreated EoE will be closely related to stricture. Ultimately, early diagnosis and treatment is the key to avoiding or delaying complications (such as stricture and severe esophageal dysfunction).

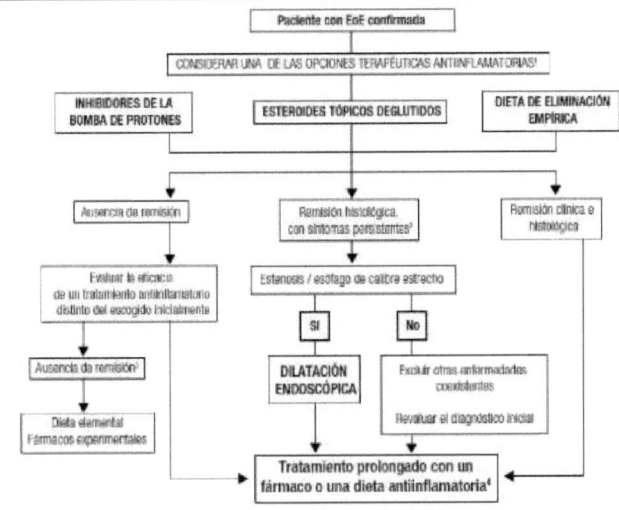

Summary

Eosinophilic esophagitis (EE) is an emerging disease characterized by a dense infiltration of the esophagus by eosinophilic leukocytes. Its main symptoms are dysphagia and frequent food impactions in the esophagus, in response to a hypersensitivity reaction to different foods or aeroallergens. The accumulation of eosinophils in the esophageal epithelium in response to local production of eosinophilotropic cytokines and chemokines has been documented in animal models and has been proposed to be in response to a TH2-type hypersensitivity reaction. The esophageal epithelium contains all the cell types necessary to develop local immunoallergic responses following CD4+ T lymphocyte stimulation. However, there is increasing evidence of the relevant role that humoral immunity plays in this disease, through the action of immunoglobulin E, mainly on mast cells. The predominance of CD8+ T lymphocytes in the inflammatory infiltrate also suggests a possible TH1 reaction in the mechanism of the disease. The proteins contained in the cytoplasmic granules of the eosinophils and activated mast cells could act on the neuromuscular components of the esophageal wall, triggering motor disturbances objectifiable by manometry that justify the esophageal symptoms.

The cause is immunological allergy and is triggered in most cases by non-IgE mediated food allergies. It is now a common disease in Europe, the United States and Australia and is emerging in South America and Asia.

In the last ten years important improvements in the algorithm of treatment of the disease include proton pump inhibitors as anti-inflammatory drugs, also appeared new topical corticosteroids specially designed for the disease. The diagnosis is clinical, endoscopic and anatomopathological. Upper endoscopy (EDA) is required to evaluate characteristic findings and to take biopsies for histological study. The update on the treatment of eosinophilic esophagitis is elimination of the diet and receiving endoscopic dilation.

Abbreviations

EoE: eosinophilic esophagitis.
EOS/CGA: high magnification field eosinophils.
GERD: gastroesophageal reflux disease.
PPI: proton pump inhibitor.

Bibliography

Arias, A., & Lucendo, A. J. (2019). Incidence and prevalence of eosinophilic oesophagitis increase continiously in adults and children in Central Spain: A 12-year population-based study. Digestive and Liver Disease, 51(1), 55-62.

Ballart, M. J., Monrroy, H., Iruretagoyena, M., Parada, A., Torres, J., & Espino, A. (2020). Eosinophilic esophagitis: diagnosis and management. Revista medica de Chile, 148(6), 831-841.

Beltran, C., Garrta, R., Espino, A., & Silva, C. (2009). Eosinophilic esophagitis: an emerging entity. Revista de otorrinolaringolog^a y cirug^a de cabeza y cuello, 69(3), 287-298.

Gori, H., Tovar, A., Ruiz, M. E., Madrid, Y., Wever, W., & Olza, M. (2010). Endoscopic-morphological findings in eosinophilic esophagitis. Gen, 64(4), 332-334.

J. Lucendo, A., 2007. Eosinophagitis Eosinofflica. [online] Medicina Clhica. Available at: < https://www.sciencedirect.com/science/article/abs/pii/S0025775307726659> [Accessed 6 December 2020].

Lucendo, A. J., Molina-Infante, J., Arias, A., von Arnim, U., Bredenoord, A. J., Bussmann, C.,.... & Miehlke, S. (2017). Guidelines on eosinophilic esophagitis: evidence-based statements and recommendations for diagnosis and management in children and adults. United European gastroenterology journal, 5(3), 335-358.

Molina-Infante, J., Corti, R., Doweck, J., & Lucendo, A. J. (2018). Therapeutic update in eosinophilic esophagitis. Acta Gastroenterol Latinoam, 48(3), 242-252.

Pierre, R., Guisande, A., Sifontes, L., Sosa, P., Ninomiya, I., Gonzalez, L., ... & Rojo, C. (2015). Diagnosis and treatment of eosinophilic esophagitis in children. Literature review and evidence-based recommendations. Working group of the Latin American Society of Pediatric Gastroenterology, Hepatology and Nutrition (SLAGHNP). Acta Gastroenterologica Latinoamericana, 45(3), 263-271.

Villann, A. J. L., & de Rezende, L. (2007). Eosinophilic esophagitis. Review of current pathophysiological and clinical concepts. Gastroenterolog^a and hepatolog^a, 30(4), 234-243.

Chapter 3
Allergic Rhinitis Dr. Roberto Galeana Rfos

Introduction

Allergic rhinitis (AR) is the most frequent respiratory disease of chronic rhinitis, it is a manifestation of hypersensitivity type 1, whose shock organ is the nasal structures, and which consists of inflammation of the nasal mucosa by an allergic reaction with the participation of mast cells, lymphocytes and eosinophils, but also of pro-inflammatory molecules (interleukins 4,5,13,17 21, leukotrienes and platelet activating factor), in addition to the spermatogenic inflammatory reaction of the adaptive response mediated by spermatogenic IgE immunoglobulin with the presence of rhinorrhea, sneezing (in salva), nasal (and ocular) pruritus, nasal obstruction and hyposmia. It can occur in any individual, at any age, race or sex, and is most commonly found in industrialized countries.

Worldwide it affects approximately 10% to 30% of the population, the prevalence is increasing, possibly related to environmental pollution and climate change.

It is common to observe that the patient's quality of life is affected in the personal, school, work and social environment. Being one of the main causes of life in relationship and school and work absenteeism. Without obviating the expenses that it represents in health and that the complications can be severe as the presentation of asthma or hearing loss especially in the pediatric age, it can generate in the infantile population dysfunctions in the attention and intellectual development.

According to the ARIA classification categorizes patients with allergic rhinitis into two types: Rhinitis allergic intermittent (RAI) and Rhinitis allergic persistent (RAP), being the same symptoms in both presentations, but differ in their duration and severity. RAI means that symptoms are present less than 4 days a week or less than 4 weeks, and RAP means that symptoms are present more than 4 days a week and for more than 4 weeks.

Classically AR has also been divided into seasonal AR and perennial AR, in relation to the dates of presentation of symptoms, in places like Mexico City due to climatic and environmental conditions perennial allergic rhinitis predominates.

Immunopathology

It should be noted that the individual who develops an allergic disease such as allergic rhinitis has a history of atopy (family inheritance) a high predisposition and susceptibility to generate the disease and that is related to exposure to aeroallergens for long periods of time, in addition to pollution, viral infections and sudden changes in temperature.

The inflammatory response of an atopic individual to allergen contact and sensitization is type 1 hypersensitivity, from the Gell and Coombs classification.

The inflammation caused in these atopic individuals is initiated by the development of events that generate allergen-specific TH2 cells that produce interleukins 4, 5, 9 and 13, which regulate the mechanisms and effector functions and induce the production of allergen-specific IgE by B lymphocytes, and whose corresponding FcERI receptors are located on the surface of the primed cells. When IgE activates the primed cell after contact with the originating anUgen, degranulation of the cell occurs, releasing preformed chemical mediators (histamine, tryptase and PAF) and the synthesis of new molecules (leukotrienes and prostaglandins), with high inflammatory activity responsible for the manifestations of AR (increased blood flow, increased vascular permeability), histamine has a local and regional action on the nasal venous and arteriolar vasculature as well as a direct effect on the central and autonomic nervous system. This allergic reaction produces vasodilation, with increased watery or mucopurulent rhinorrhea, due to stimulation of the sensitive nerve endings, giving rise to local and regional pruritus and alterations in the autonomic nervous system. Therefore, as rhinitis progresses, sensitization becomes more intense and the picture of allergic rhinitis intensifies.

Classical presentation

The classic symptoms of allergic rhinitis are the rhinorrhea that accompanies sneezing, which is usually called in a series because of the sequential form in which it occurs, unilateral or bilateral nasal obstruction and nasal itching (ocular, palatine, pharyngeal and otic), the prevalence of each of the symptoms depends on the duration of the symptomatic phase, in the acute phase it is common to find sneezing followed by hyaline anterior rhinorrhea and unilateral or bilateral nasal obstruction and in the chronic phase, the latter is the most rebellious to treatment. In the chronic phase it is frequent to find besides nasal obstruction, frontal headache, in projection of maxillary paranasal sinuses, hyposmia and anosmia, also behavioral or learning disorders; in the case of children, hypoacusia, rhinolalia and asthma. Lately, it has been found in patients with chronic allergic rhinitis and it is increasing the recurrent epistaxis.

On physical examination, we can find, depending on the time of evolution of allergic rhinitis, a pale nasal mucosa, edematous, shiny, with anterior aqueous rhinorrhea forming hyaline bridges or posterior discharge or drip, turbinate hypertrophy, nasal voice, pain on palpation in maxillary and frontal sinuses, cosmetic changes such as allergic furrow (a transverse fold at the border of the cartiliginous and bony portion of the nose) caused by intense and continuous scratching by the patient and which, when performed by the patient, resembles an allergic salute due to the movements, Dennie-Morgan's lmeas which are double folded furrows in the lower eyelids also caused by scratching due to ocular itching when the damage is regionalized, dark circles under the eyes caused by local venous stasis, adenoid fascies in children, oral respiration, rhinolalia, dry cough, odynophagia and hypertrophy of the tonsils. In chronic cases of allergic rhinitis and where air pollution is also accentuated, we find a pale nasal mucosa, but with intense dryness, bilateral nasal obstruction, dry cough, and nocturnal oral respiration.

Diagnostic, laboratory and cabinet

The diagnosis should be oriented not only to control the nasal symptoms of the individual but also to the search for the cause of the symptomatology of the disease. This is possible through an adequate clinical history of the patient, where we can look for predisposing antecedents (family atopy), triggering factors (viral infections, environmental pollution), personal pathological antecedents (atopic dermatitis, food allergy, asthma), season and frequency in which the symptoms occur.

The usual studies to be performed are blood biometry, where we can find an increase in eosinophils, although not finding them does not rule out AR. Cytology of nasal mucus, the search for eosinophils in nasal secretion is a good parameter, however the negativity of these does not rule out AR. Nasal discharge culture if an infectious component is suspected. Dosage of total IgE, is not a pathognomonic parameter, since it can be found in high concentrations in parasitic processes, however it is convenient to have serum levels as it is a helpful data. X-rays of paranasal sinuses in cadwell, watters and lateral projections, CT of paranasal sinuses is helpful when there is suspicion of paranasal complications. And cutaneous tests with specific aeroallergens, are performed to verify the clinical impression that has been obtained to the interrogation and clinical exploration, for this standardized allergenic extracts are used and that are related to the environment where the patient lives, the most used intradomiciliary aeroallergens are house dust mites, and among the extradomiciliary pollen and fungal spores. Positive results indicate that the patient is atopic and help to find the aeroallergen responsible (specific aeroallergen IgE).

Differential diagnosis/ complications

Infectious, idiopathic or vasomotor, occupational, chemical/irritative, drug-induced, non-allergic rhinitis with eosinophilia, hormonal, atrophic, anatomic, nasal polyposis, vasculitis rhinitis, and autoimmune rhinitis.

One of the most frequent complications is sinusitis, rhinitis medicamentosa.

Treatment

Treatment of AR can be done through three pillars:

First pillar environmental control is possible when the cause of the disease is known, by avoiding exposure to aeroallergens.

Second pillar symptom control, pharmacological control with antihistamines and ICS.

Third pillar specific control, control with specific subcutaneous or sublingual aeroallergen immunotherapy.

However, before going deeper into these aspects, it is necessary to take into account the evidence presented in the ARIA guide for a global evaluation of AR.

Bibliography

Amerigo A, Sanchez M, Barbarroja J, Alvarez-Mon M. Allergic rhinitis. Medicine. 2017; 12(30):1757-66

Brozek J, Bousquet J, Agache I, Agarwa A, Bachert C, Bosnic-Anticevich S, et al. Allergic Rhinitis and its Impact on Asthma (ARIA) guidelines-2016 revision. J Allergy Clin Immunol. 2016; 140:950-9.

Rodriguez-Santos O, Nancy del Valle-Monteagudo N. Immunotherapy with industrial extracts of house mites in children under 5 years of age with rhinitis and asthma. VacciMonitor 2018; 27(2):61 -66 www.vaccimonitor.finlay.edu.cu

Chapter 4

Allergic rhinitis and sleep apnea Dr. Olimpio Rodriguez Santos & Zuriel Flores Silveiro

Introduction

RA is one of the diseases that can be accompanied by sleep disorders, causing interruption of oxygen uptake during breathing, and consequently, in severe cases, resulting in the death of neurons. The function of breathing allows the cells to obtain the oxygen they need to survive, and the absence of this process causes death. This is why for a long time it was considered the moment in which we stop breathing as the exact time to die. It is an indispensable thing that is necessary, even when the level of consciousness is altered or when we sleep. Sometimes during sleep, for a few seconds, alterations occur that hinder this vital process.

Sleep and its phases

The Global Sleep Observatory (GSO) defines sleep as a complex physiological phenomenon, fundamental to human health. It is a universal process in the animal kingdom and is a basic need of our organism that allows us to rest and recover physically and mentally. It is characterized by changes in physiological activity and a reduced response to external stimuli.
The relationship between the quality of sleep and the body's ability to recover from certain serious and highly prevalent diseases has been scientifically proven. Likewise, sleep problems can be related to important complications and certain diseases, such as major depression, myocardial infarction, fibromyalgia, rheumatoid arthritis, osteoarthritis or Alzheimer's disease, among others.

Sleep and wakefulness are two states of brain activity that follow each other in a cyclical manner. According to the electrical activity of the brain, there are different phases of sleep:
Phase 1: drowsiness
Phase 2: superficial sleep
Phase 3: deep sleep

REM Phase: (Rapid Eye Movement). It is considered unsynchronized sleep. The REM or REM (Rapid Eye Movement) phase is one of the most important phases of sleep. It is characterized by the presence of a high brain activity, which can be visible in the realization of rapid and constant eye movements. Normally, adult nighttime sleep is organized in 5-6 cycles of 60-90 minutes. The efficiency, distribution and overall percentage of the different phases of sleep give information about the duration and structure of the sleep. The adequacy of these parameters to the described values of normality is used to evaluate the quality of sleep. The study of sleep quality is an objective of this chapter especially when disorders such as sleep apnea occur in patients with AR.

Breathing disorders during sleep

Respiratory sleep disorders are understood as the set of alterations that occur during the period of sleep in which there is insufficient ventilation or breathing or a change in the respiratory rhythm. Sleep disorders are conditions that cause changes in the way you sleep. A sleep disorder can affect health, safety, and quality of life. Lack of sleep can affect the ability to drive safely and increase the risk of other health problems.

Most of the time, these are disorders in which apneas appear, or brief periods in which the patient stops breathing for at least ten seconds and usually generates a partial awakening to be able to inhale and receive oxygen. There is also another associated concept, called hypoapnea, in which the subject does not stop breathing, but the amount of air entering the body is greatly reduced by becoming more shallow breathing.

These disorders often lead to nocturnal awakenings, which are mostly not consciously perceived, and are often associated with the onset of snoring. They often have consequences, perhaps the most visible being the difficulty in maintaining a continuous and restful sleep, which can result in the appearance of daytime sleepiness, fatigue and difficulty concentrating. You may also suffer from relationship problems, such as discomfort and conflict with bed partners.

Breathing disorders during sleep can have a number of serious health consequences if they are not treated correctly. They can have very harmful effects on the cardiovascular system, constituting a risk factor for heart disease. And is that the obstruction of the air passage generates pulmonary hypertension and an overload in the right ventricle of the heart, part of the heart responsible for sending blood to the lungs for re-oxygenation. This can lead to a greater likelihood of arrhythmias, angina pectoris and even myocardial infarction.

It can also have cognitive effects, as it hinders the maintenance and rhythmicity of sleep cycles and, in addition, the presence of repeated micro-anoxias can lead to the death of groups of neurons as mentioned above. In children, it can also lead to growth and developmental delays, as well as increased insulin resistance or other metabolic problems. It has also been observed to be detrimental to patients with diabetes and neuromuscular disorders. The US National Library of Medicine documents more than 100 different sleep and wakefulness disorders. Insomnia is one of the most common and, according to the OGS, in Spain, between 20% and 30% of the population suffers from it. The other most common is the obstructive sleep apnea syndrome (OSAS) or sleep apnea, which, due to its high prevalence (between five and seven million Spaniards suffer from it) and the risks it entails (illness, death, and death from sleep apnea), is one of the most common sleep disorders in Spain.

cardiovascular disease, hypertension, increased risk of mortality and even cancer), it is considered a public health problem.

Types of Sleep Breathing Disorders

There are several phenomena that could be considered sleep breathing disorders with different levels of impact on the individual who suffers from them. Some of the most common are:

Obstructive sleep apnea

Obstructive sleep apnea is a disorder in which one suffers, during sleep, from obstruction of the upper airways, despite continuing to perform the action of breathing. The respiratory rate increases in an attempt to receive the air that is lacking for normal breathing.

Non-conscious awakenings and micro-awakenings during sleep are frequent, although the subject eventually wakes up to the contraction of the muscles linked to breathing, in search of oxygen. This may occur several times during the night.

One of the most frequent symptoms is the presence of irregular and high intensity snoring, in addition to the awakenings caused by the search for air by the organism. It is not uncommon to experience vivid dreams and high levels of night sweats. During the day there is usually fatigue, lack of strength, memory problems and decreased sexual appetite. Arrhythmias are common and can facilitate the onset of severe heart problems.

Central Sleep Apnea
Central sleep apneas occur when the airways are not obstructed allowing air to pass through, but there is a decrease in airflow. The problem itself is that the body does not make the effort to breathe normally. There is an interruption of airflow due to reduced or absent respiratory effort. Problem derived from a cardiac or cerebral alteration, and there may be numerous possible causes behind it. Unlike other apneas and sleep disorders, snoring is not common, and may not even be detected directly. What is perceived is the presence of daytime fatigue, nocturnal awakenings caused by the sensation of drowning and sometimes fear of sleeping due to these sensations.

Mixed sleep apnea
It is a respiratory disorder during sleep that combines the characteristics of the two previous ones: the respiratory problem begins with a central apnea in which the effort to breathe is greatly diminished, but when it will return to normal rhythms appears a real obstruction of the respiratory tract that usually generates the awakening of the subject.

Upper Airway Resistance Syndrome
A syndrome of lesser severity than the others in which there is no decrease in the levels of oxygen received. This disorder is characterized by the presence of awakenings during sleep, without the occurrence of an episode of apnea. The problem in this case seems to be linked to an increase in the effort made to breathe in. Intense snoring usually appears as a result of this effort. It also tends to generate daytime sleepiness.

Hypoventilation Shdromes
These shdromes are characterized because, unlike apneas, there is no period

of time in which there is a complete cessation of breathing. They are smdromes in which the subject who suffers them has some kind of deficiency in the respiratory system that does not reach a sufficient level of air to the body, usually being shallow breathing. Less oxygen reaches the brain and there is an increase in the levels of carbon dioxide in the blood.

It is not infrequent that snoring appears, and like the previous ones it usually causes fatigue, memory problems and some nocturnal awakenings. We talk about shdromes because there are several that could be included in this category, such as the Ondina shdrome.

Ondina syndrome, technically called congenital central hypoventilation syndrome (CCHS) or primary alveolar hypoventilation, and colloquially Ondina's curse, is a respiratory disorder that is fatal if left untreated. Sufferers typically suffer from cardiorespiratory arrest during sleep. CCHS is either congenital or developed due to severe neurological trauma to the brain stem. Diagnosis may be delayed due to variations in the severity of manifestations or lack of awareness in the medical community, especially in milder cases. There are also cases where the diagnosis is made in adulthood and middle age, although the symptoms are usually evident in retrospect. Again, lack of awareness in the medical community may cause this delay. This is a very rare and severe form of central nervous system failure, involving a congenital failure of autonomic breathing control. Approximately 1 in 200,000 live births have the symptoms. In 2006, there were only about 200 known cases worldwide. In all cases, episodes of apnea occur during sleep, but in some patients, at the more severe end of the spectrum, apnea also occurs during wakefulness.

General Symptomatology

Sleep apnea is a common disorder in which breathing is interrupted or becomes very shallow. These interruptions can last from a few seconds to minutes and can occur more than 30 times per hour.

The most important symptom is the continuous snoring which then stops and a pause in breathing may appear. When there is only one respiratory stop during the night, it is not possible to affirm that there is a pathology, but if the pauses are continuous, it is a very important sign of this disease.

The arrival of a new study from the University of Pennsylvania shows that the symptoms caused by sleep apnea can be reduced by reducing the fat on the tongue.

In 2014, the journal Sleep, published the first study that found a relationship between the size and fat deposits of the tongue and apnea. The work was carried out with 90 adults suffering from obesity in addition to the sleep disorder and 31 obese controls without it. All subjects underwent magnetic resonance imaging (MRI) of the upper respiratory tract. Volumetric reconstruction algorithms were used to study the size and distribution of fat deposits in the upper respiratory tract and tongue.

The researchers proposed that, in addition to increasing the volume of the tongue, the increased fat could affect the function of the muscles that attach the tongue to the bone, preventing these muscles from positioning the tongue farther away from the airway.

On the other hand, we are seeing patients with glaucoma associated with apnea and the relationship is very clear. When there is apnea, the oxygen concentration drops, and this fact, which accumulates over the years, has consequences and one of them is visual health. Other consequences are cardiovascular and brain health.

Causes of the appearance of these disorders

The reasons for the appearance of some kind of respiratory disorder during sleep can be multiple, both genetic and environmental. Alterations of a biological and genetic nature can be found in the presence of cranial malformations or in hypertrophies of organs such as the tongue or the tonsils, or in different smdromes and diseases, both genetic and acquired.

One of the most relevant controllable risk factors is obesity. Increased fatty tissue, especially around the throat, can exert weight and pressure on the airways, making it difficult for air to pass through. Obstruction and impairment of the airways can also contribute to the development or maintenance of a respiratory disorder during sleep, such as smoking. Allergies are also a possible reason for its appearance as in the particular case of AR that is developed in this chapter.

They can also be linked (as in the case of central apneas) or derive from the presence of a cardiopaUa or brain injury that may be derived from infections, cardiovascular or cerebrovascular accidents, tumours, respiratory diseases or cranioencephalic trauma.

Some of the signs and symptoms of sleep disorders include excessive daytime sleepiness, irregular breathing, or increased movement during sleep. Other signs and symptoms include irregular sleep and wake cycle and difficulty falling asleep. There are many different types of sleep disorders. Often, they are grouped into categories that explain why they happen or how they affect you. Sleep disorders can also be classified according to behaviors, problems with natural sleep-wake cycles, breathing problems, difficulty falling asleep, or how sleepy you feel during the day. In another classification, some common types of sleep disorders include:

- Insomnia, which is difficulty falling asleep or staying asleep during the night.
- Sleep apnea, which is having abnormal breathing patterns while asleep.
- Restless legs syndrome, a type of sleep movement disorder. This syndrome, also called Willis-Ekbom disease, causes an uncomfortable sensation and an urge to move your legs when you are trying to fall asleep.
- Narcolepsy, a condition characterized by extreme sleepiness during the day and suddenly falling asleep during the day.

Causes of sleep disorders

In the case of insomnia, anxiety, hyperthyroidism, psychiatric illnesses or those that produce pain are the most common causes.

In hypersomnia, the causes may be associated with anxiety or severe depression, hypnotic abuse or sleep apnea.

Sleep disorders due to psychiatric illnesses

a. Psychosis.
b. Mood disorders.
c. Anxiety disorders.
d. Drug addictions.

Sleep disorders due to neurological disorders:

a. Neurodegenerative diseases.
b. Dementias.
c. Epilepsies.
d. Cranioencephalic traumas.
e. Headaches.

Sleep disorders due to other medical causes

a. Chronic obstructive pulmonary disease (COPD).
b. Fibromyalgia.
c. Asthma.

d. Obesity.
   e. Gastrointestinal diseases.
   f. Respiratory diseases.
   g. Kidney diseases.

In RA more than 50% of patients have sleep disorders and one in five suffers excessive daytime sleepiness due to this cause, according to the study 'Somniaar', which has had the scientific endorsement of the Spanish Society of Allergology and Clinical Immunology (SEAIC) and the Spanish Society of Otorhinolaryngology (SEORL).

In the case of a patient with suspected AR, it is necessary to make the definitive diagnosis as described in chapter 3, also considering the possibility that it is accompanied by sleep apnea or another related disorder.

Diagnostic

Questioning of the patient or family member, with emphasis on nocturnal snoring and physical examination, leads to an evaluation for signs and symptoms and sleep history, which may be possible with the help of someone who sleeps in the same room as the patient. A proper evaluation usually involves nightly monitoring of breathing and other bodily functions while the patient sleeps in a sleep center or appropriate sleep room. Another option is to test at night at home for sleep apnea.

Sleep apnea testing

The main tests for sleep apnea include home sleep testing and overnight polysomnography.

Home Sleep Test.

These tests usually measure heart rate, blood oxygen levels, air flow, and breathing patterns. There are also several devices available to study breathing. One of these, the ApneaLink Air device (Fig. 4-1) is indicated for use by health care providers to aid in the diagnosis of sleep-disordered breathing.

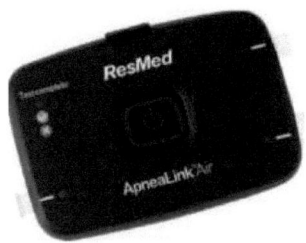
Fig. 4-1. ApneaLink Air device records the following patient data: nasal airflow, snoring, blood oxygen saturation, pulse, and respiratory effort during sleep.

If the results are abnormal, therapy may be prescribed without further testing. However, portable monitoring devices do not detect all cases of sleep apnea, so a polysomnogram may be recommended even if the initial results are normal.

Nocturnal polysomnography.
Several pieces of equipment are available for overnight polysomnography, one of which is attached to the patient to monitor heart, lung and brain activity, breathing patterns, arm and leg movements, and blood oxygen levels while the person sleeps. In polysomnography, sleep phases and cycles are monitored to determine if, when, and why sleep patterns are interrupted.
The normal process of falling asleep begins with a phase of sleep called non-rapid eye movement sleep (NMOR). During this phase, brain waves, as recorded on an electroencephalogram (EEG), slow down considerably.
The eyes do not move from side to side rapidly during NMOR sleep, unlike in the later phases of sleep. After an hour or two of NMOR sleep, brain activity picks up again, and rapid eye movement (REM) sleep begins. Most dreams occur during REM sleep.
You normally go through several sleep cycles in one night, with NMOR and REM sleep cycles lasting about 90 minutes. Sleep disorders can disrupt this sleep process.
Polysomnography is recommended when suspected:
- Sleep apnea or other sleep-related breathing disorder. In this disorder, breathing stops and starts repeatedly during sleep.
- Periodic leg movement disorder. In this sleep disorder, the legs involuntarily flex and extend during sleep. This disorder is sometimes associated with restless legs syndrome.
- Narcolepsy. With this disorder, you experience overwhelming

sleepiness and sudden sleep attacks during the day.
- REM sleep behavior disorder. This sleep disorder consists of acting out dreams while the individual sleeps.
- Unusual behaviors during sleep. These are activities that are out of the ordinary during sleep, such as walking, moving around a lot, or making rhythmic movements.
- Unexplained chronic insomnia. When there are constant problems falling asleep or staying asleep.

If you have obstructive sleep apnea, you may be referred to an Otolaryngologist to rule out a blockage in the nose or throat. It may be necessary to refer to a cardiologist or neurologist for evaluation in case of central sleep apnea.

Sleep Apnea-Hypopnea Syndrome (SAHS)
According to the definition of the Spanish Sleep Group, SAHS is characterized by the appearance of recurrent episodes of airflow limitation during sleep, as a consequence of an anatomical-functional alteration of the upper airway that leads to its collapse, causing decreases in oxyhemoglobin saturation and micro-awakenings leading to non-restorative sleep, excessive daytime sleepiness, neuropsychiatric, respiratory and cardiac disorders.

Classification of SAHS
Broadbent 1877, Mackenzie 1880. Guillerminault et al. recognized it as a chronic entity in 1976. The International Classification of Sleep Disorders (ISCD-2) distinguishes respiratory sleep disorders from non-respiratory sleep disorders. In the first group it establishes three main categories:
1. Obstructive Sleep Apnea Hypoapnea Obstructive Sleep Apnea Syndrome (OSAHS).
2. Central Sleep Apnea Syndrome (SACS).
3. Sleep Alveolar Hyperventilation Syndrome (SH).
4. Others include nocturnal asthma, COPD sleep disturbances, etc.

OSAHS in children
OSAHS in children can be associated with health problems, which highlight the need for early diagnosis and treatment. This pathology can lead to brain dysfunctions with behavioral disorders and learning deficits if left untreated.

OSAHS may be associated with AR in children and adults.

Allergic rhinitis as seen from its impact on asthma [ARIA].

The Allergic Rhinitis and its Impact on Asthma (ARIA) initiative was started during a World Health Organization (WHO) workshop in 1999 and published in 2001. AR is one of the most common diseases worldwide and generally persists throughout life. The prevalence of self-reported AR has been estimated to be 2% - 25% in children and 1% - 40% in adults.

The burden and costs of RA are substantial: it reduces quality of life, quality of sleep, cognitive function; causing irritability and fatigue. RA is associated with decreased school and work performance.

ARIA 2001

In ARIA 2001 the AR was classified as:

Seasonal allergic rhinitis (SAR; most often caused by outdoor allergens, such as pollens or molds)

Perennial allergic rhinitis (PAR) is most often caused by indoor allergens such as house dust mites, molds, cockroaches and animal dander.

Occupational allergic rhinitis.

Occupational allergic rhinitis is due to allergens present in the workplace: flour, latex, tropical woods, detergents, mites, laboratory animals, among others.

With few exceptions, studies refer to SAR and PAR and enroll patients based on the offending allergen such as pollen, house dust mites, or both.

ARIA 2008

The classic nasal symptoms of RA are nasal itching, sneezing, runny nose and nasal congestion.

Allergic rhinoconjunctivitis is associated with itching and redness of the eyes and tearing. Other symptoms include itching of the roof of the mouth, postnasal drip and cough.

ARIA 2010

ARIA 2010 was the first evidence-based guideline in allergy to follow the recommendations, approach to development and evaluation (GRADE). It summarized the potential benefits and harms underlying the recommendations, as well as assumptions about values and preferences that influenced the strength and direction of the recommendations.

In 2014, the ARIA review was found to rank first in the rigor of development and quality of AR management guideline reporting.

ARIA 2016

The recommendations in the 2016 ARIA update apply directly to patients with moderate to severe RA. They may be less applicable to the treatment of patients with mild RA who often do not seek medical help and manage their symptoms themselves with medications available in other conditions.

The recent survey conducted in the 4 countries of the Southeast Asian Nations (ASEAN) has identified the need to strengthen awareness of the use of ARIA guidelines among PHC professionals. Adherence to ARIA guidelines, choice of appropriate treatment option, and prioritization of factors that increase patient adherence can contribute to better management of AR outcomes at that level of health care.

Strength of recommendation
Strong recommendation

For patients:
Most patients in this situation burn the recommended course of action, and only a small proportion would not.
For doctors:
Most patients should receive the intervention. Adherence to a strong recommendation could be used as a quality criterion or performance indicator.
For health care policy makers: The recommendation can be adopted as a policy or performance measure in most situations.

Conditional recommendation

For patients: Most patients in this situation burn the suggested course of action, but many would not.
For clinicians: Recognize that different options will be appropriate for individual patients and that you should help each patient arrive at a management decision consistent with his or her values and preferences. Decision aids may be useful in helping patients make decisions consistent with their values and preferences.

For those responsible for health care policy formulation: Policy formulation will require substantial debate and participation of various stakeholders.

Limitations of the evidence

The available evidence has important limitations:

(1) selective measurement and reporting of outcomes (e.g., few studies adequately measure and report quality of life, which is the most important outcome in patients with RA,

(2) selection of patients for clinical trials that may not adequately represent patients seen in primary care,

(3) failure to distinguish between patients with different age or severity of symptoms (lack of adequate stratification), thus limiting the applicability and generalizability of the research results.

Clinical diagnosis of sleep apnea and RA

The clinical diagnosis of sleep apnea is given, in the first instance, by a patient who presents oral breathing accompanied by snoring. The patient may have a family history of similar symptoms. On interrogation it is detected that breathing is interrupted while the person sleeps.

It has been known for years that being overweight influences the number of apneas and that the fat accumulated in the oropharynx (tongue, posterior pillars) favours snoring or this relaxation.

People who are overweight, have a peculiar facial morphology (short and wide neck) and also those who have retrognathia mandibularis (small jaw set back) are more at risk for the disorder and, even if they are thin, may have the disorder. Apneas are also seen in children if they have tonsillar hypertrophy. Anything that hinders the passage of air in and out of the lungs through abnormal oropharyngeal structures can cause these apneas.

The question about drowsiness has to be asked: ^In the absence of stimuli to keep you alert, do you feel sleepy? If the answer is yes, there is pathological sleepiness and this happens if we are in the middle of the morning watching the clock and fall asleep. If there is drowsiness while driving or in a meeting in the middle of the morning, we have a disorder. In advanced situations are people who during the night have a dry mouth, drink a lot of water or go to the bathroom many times. It is important to keep in mind that diastolic arterial hypertension (hypertension) is a symptom that, together with snoring and drowsiness, can lead to the suspicion of apneas.

The clinical diagnosis of AR is based on personal and family history of atopy and on the classic nasal symptoms of AR given by nasal itching, sneezing, rhinorrhea and nasal congestion. Prick test confirms the etiological diagnosis in most cases.

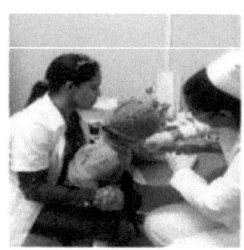

Fig. 4-2. Prick test in AR. Skin test that allows to confirm the cause and consequently apply allergy vaccines as specific treatment. In early life, a well performed test can prevent future complications and achieve a better quality of life for the child and the family.

Evidence-based treatment of AR

ARIA addresses 6 questions about AR treatment

1. Should a combination of oral H1-antihistamine and intranasal corticosteroid be used versus intranasal corticosteroids alone for the treatment of AR?
2. Whether a combination of intranasal H1-antihistamine and intranasal corticosteroid vs. intranasal corticosteroids alone for the treatment of AR?
3. Should a combination of an intranasal H1 antihistamine and an intranasal corticosteroid be used versus an intranasal H1 antihistamine alone for the treatment of AR?
4. Should a leukotriene receptor antagonist be used versus an oral H1-antihistamine for the treatment of AR?
5. Should an intranasal H1 antihistamine be used versus an intranasal corticosteroid for the treatment of AR?
6. Should an intranasal H1-antihistamine be used versus an oral H1-antihistamine for the treatment of AR?

Table, 1. Recommendations

Question 1: ^Should a combination of an oral H1 antihistamine (OAH) and an intranasal corticosteroid (INCS) vs. INCS alone be used to treat increased AR without consequence?

Recommendation.	Assumed values and preferences	Explanations and considerations
Recommendation 1A: In patients with SAR, we suggest combining an INCS with an OAH or an INCS alone (conditional recommendation with low certainty of evidence). Recommendation 1B: In patients with PAR, an INCS alone is suggested instead of a combination of an INCS with an OAH (conditional recommendation - very low certainty of evidence).	The ARIA guideline panel recognized that the choice of treatment would depend primarily on patient preference, local availability, and cost of treatment. Panel members presumed that, in most situations, the potential net benefit would not justify expending additional resources.	Recommendation is conditional, and therefore different options will be appropriate for different patients. The additional cost of OAH is not great and/or patient values and preferences differ from those assumed by the guideline panel members, a combination therapy may be a solution in patients whose symptoms are not well controlled with an INCS alone, those with pronounced ocular symptoms.

Seasonal Allergic Rhinitis (SAR) Perennial Allergic Rhinitis (PAR)

Question 2: ^Should a combination of an intranasal H 1 antihistamine (INAH) and INCS vs. an INCS alone be used for the treatment of AR?

Recommendation 2A: In patients with SAR, we suggest a combination of an INCS with an INAH or an INCS alone (conditional recommendation - moderate certainty of evidence).	Panel members recognized that the choice of treatment will depend primarily on patient preference and local availability and cost of treatment. At treatment initiation (approximately the first 2 weeks), a combination of an INCS with an INAH may act more quickly than an INCS alone and therefore may be preferred by some patients.	This is a conditional recommendation, and therefore different options will be appropriate for different patients. In settings where the additional cost of combination therapy is not great and/or patients value the potential benefits more than any increased risk of adverse effects, combination therapy may be a reasonable option.

Question 3: ^Should a combination of an INAH and an INCS be used vs. an INAH alone for the treatment of AR?

| Recommendation 3A: In patients with SAR, we suggest a combination of an INCS with an INAH rather than an INAH alone (conditional recommendation - low certainty of evidence). | This recommendation places a higher value on additional symptom reduction and quality of life improvement with combination therapy compared to INAH alone. It reduces the value by avoiding additional cost (resource expenditure). | Recommendation is conditional, and therefore different options will be appropriate for different patients. In settings where the additional cost of combination therapy is great, an alternative option (i.e., INAH alone) may be equally reasonable. |

Question 4: ^Should a leukotriene receptor antagonist (LTRA) be used versus an OAH for the treatment of AR?

| Recommendation 4A: In patients with SAR, we suggest an LTRA or an OAH (conditional recommendation - moderate certainty of evidence). | Panel members acknowledged that the choice of LTRA or OAH will depend on patient preference and the local availability and cost of specific medications. | Some patients with AR who have concomitant exercise-induced or aspirin-exacerbated asthma may benefit from LTRA rather than OAH. However, this recommendation applies to the treatment of AR but not to the treatment of asthma which should be adequately treated according to asthma treatment guidelines. |
| Recommendation 4B: In patients with PAR, we suggest an OAH rather than an LTRA (conditional recommendation - low certainty of evidence). | This recommendation places a higher value on the possibly greater improvement in symptoms and quality of life with LTRA. It places a lower value on the possible increased risk of drowsiness. | Conditional recommendation, and therefore different options will be appropriate for different patients depending on their preferences for symptom reduction versus avoiding the risk of adverse effects. This may be more important for patients with PAR than those with SAR because they may be able to use those medications for longer periods of time. Some patients with AR and concomitant asthma, especially exercise-induced and/or aspirin-exacerbated respiratory disease, may benefit from an LTRA rather than an OAH. However, this recommendation applies to the treatment of AR but not asthma. |

Question 5: ^Should an INAH vs. an INCS be used to treat AR?

Recommendation 5A: In patients with SAR, we suggest an INCS instead of an INAH (conditional recommendation - moderate certainty of evidence).	This recommendation places a higher value on the likely small but greater reduction in symptoms and improvement in quality of life with an INCS compared to an INAH and a lower value on avoiding the higher cost of treatment with an INCS in many jurisdictions.	This is a conditional recommendation, and therefore different options will be appropriate for different patients. Physicians should assist each patient in arriving at a decision consistent with their values and preferences, taking into account local availability and costs.
Recommendation 5B: In PAR, we suggest an INCS instead of an INAH (conditional recommendation - low certainty of evidence).	This recommendation places a higher value on probably a greater reduction in nasal symptoms with INCS compared to an INAH, although the difference is probably small. It places a lower value on avoiding a higher cost of treatment with an INCS.	Recommendation is conditional, and therefore different options will be appropriate for different patients. Physicians should assist each patient in arriving at a decision consistent with his or her values and preferences, taking into account local availability and costs.

Question 6: ^Should an INAH be used versus an OAH for the treatment of AR?

Recommendation 6A: In patients with SAR, we suggest an INAH or OAH (conditional recommendation - low certainty of evidence).	The members of the panel acknowledged that the choice of treatment will depend primarily on local availability and the cost of treatment.	This is a recommendation conditional, and therefore different options will be appropriate for different patients. Physicians should help each patient arrive at a decision consistent with his or her preferences, considering local availability, coverage and costs.
Recommendation 6B: In patients with PAR, we suggest an INAH or OAH (conditional recommendation - very low certainty of evidence).	Panel members acknowledged that the choice of treatment will depend primarily on local availability and the cost of treatment.	This is a conditional recommendation, and therefore different options will be appropriate for different patients. Physicians should help each patient arrive at a decision

		consistent with their preferences, taking into account local availability, coverage and costs.

Taken and modified from: Brozek et al. Allergic Rhinitis and its Impact on Asthma (ARIA) guidelines-2016 revision. J Allergy Clin Immunol 2017 Volume 140, Number 4:950-958
INAH, intranasal H 1 -antihistamine; INCS, intranasal corticosteroid; LTRA, leukotriene receptor antagonist; OAH, oral H 1 -antihistamine.

Allergen Specific Immunotherapy (ASIT).

The treatment of AR, in patients with sleep apnea, using ITAE is still novel, among other reasons because, although ITAE is a common procedure in AR, the possibility that it may be related to patients with sleep disorders is not always investigated.

However, from the PHC it is possible to make the diagnosis of both, and in a short time to achieve a better quality of life. To do this it is important to review some indicators considered analysis indexes that are recorded by the ApneaLink Air device.

AHI (apnea-hypopnea index): average number of all types of apnea (indeterminate, central, mixed, obstructive) and hypopneas per hour during the evaluation period. Events are also displayed individually in the apnea and hypopnea index fields. If the measured value exceeds the normal range, it will be "framed".

IR (risk indicator):

The risk indicator (RI) is calculated as follows:

IR = score expressed as the sum of the AHI + Lf/LR score

Points calculated from the AHI:

AHI x 1 h = number of points (e.g. AHI = 5/h x 1 h = 5 points) where h is the evaluation period.

Lf/LR Score:

Number of points = 10 x (0.8 x Lf + 1.2 x LR) / Fi where:
- AHI = apnoea-hypopnoea index
- Lf = number of flow-limited breaths without snoring
- LR = number of flow-limited and snoring breaths
- Fi = total number of breaths

If the measured value exceeds the normal range, it will be "framed".

% of flow-limited breaths without R (Lf): percentage of all flow-limited breaths without snoring, relative to the sum of all breaths.

% Flow Restricted Breaths with R (LR): The percentage of all flow-limited breaths with snoring, relative to the sum of all breaths. An LR is only assessed if a simultaneous snoring event occurs that exceeds 30% of the duration of flow restriction.

The data below appears in the report if pulse oximetry is performed.

SpO2 assessment period: The SpO2 assessment period is the saturation time recorded excluding artifacts, sensor failures, and the first 10 minutes of recording, marked by the start of the assessment saturation event.

IDO (oxygen desaturation index):

This is an average value that shows the number of desaturations within the SpO2 evaluation period.

If the measured value exceeds the normal range, it will be "framed".

The ApneaLink Air system includes:
1	Dispositive ApneaLink Air	5	Oximeter
2	Stress sensor	6	Disposable digital oximeter sensor*.
3	Belt	7	Reusable Digital Oximeter Sensor*
4	Oximeter belt clamp*.	8	Nasal Cannula
		9	Handbag (not shown)

This item may only be available as an accessory in some countries.

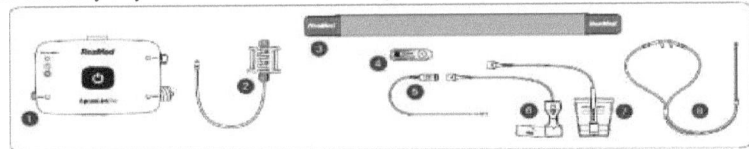

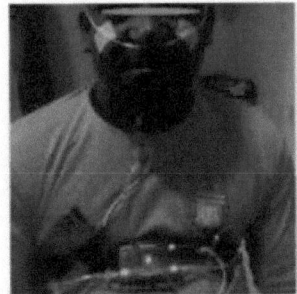 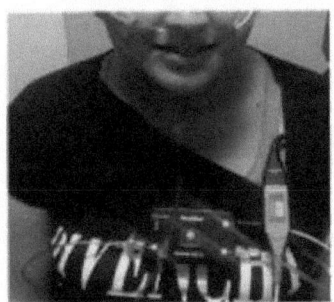

AB

Fig. 4-2.A. Patient with severe OSAHS diagnosed by the clinic and pathological CRP. B moderate clinical and CRP between normal limits.

Corresponds to Fig 4-2 A. Patients with severe OSAHS diagnosed by the clinic and pathologic CRP. Note the IAH, IR and IDO indices.

Corresponds to Fig 4-2B. Patient with AR and clinical suspicion of OSAHS with normal CRP.

Children with RA sensitized to house mites have a high probability of having sleep apnea hypopnea-ostructive sleep apnea syndrome (HOSAS) that disappears or improves with AITI.

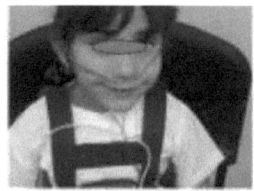 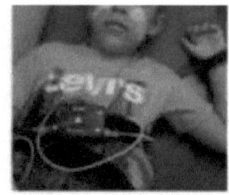
CD
Fig. 4-3. C and D. ApneaLink Air disositive study of two suspected sleep apnea patients.

The study with the ApneaLink Air device can confirm the diagnosis and also serves as a follow-up test to assess the evolution. In the Preventive Allergy Service, the study is carried out in suspected cases and 236 patients between 8 and 70 years of age have been included in the first study.
102 cases (43.2%) defined as those with mouth breathing and snoring and 134 controls (56.7%) with neither mouth breathing nor snoring.
Cardiorespiratory polygraph (CRP) was performed using the ApneaLink AirTM automatic event tagging device (Resmed Corp., RFA).
In the Prick test, the mean size of the wheal was 5.9 mm in cases (p=0.02). The apnea-hypopnea index (AHI) was positive in 129 patients (54.6%); of them, 97 cases (41.1%) and 32 controls (13.5%).
Patients with AHI>20/h predominated in cases with 21 individuals (8.8%) (p=0.048). The sensitivity of CRP was 95.10%, its specificity 76.12%. The positive and negative predictive values were 75.19% and 95.33% respectively. The positive likelihood ratio was estimated at 3.98 and the negative likelihood ratio at 0.06.
Patients with OSAHS in cases and controls presented an increase with a predominance for cases (p=0.002). The PCR with the ApneaLink device allows the diagnosis of OSAHS in AR.

In a second study 326 patients were selected in consecutive order of attendance to the consultation, taking into account the criteria: >5 years with AR, suspicion of OSA and skin test with mites: *Dermatophagoides pteronyssinus*, *Dermatophagoides siboney* and *Blomia tropicalis*, produced in: "Centro Nacional de Biopreparados" of Cuba. All received specific allergy immunotherapy (ITAE) for ^10 months and PCR was performed before and after ITAE.
PCR was performed using the ApneaLink AirTM automated event tagging

system (Resmed Corp., RFA), validated for studying sleep disorders at home. The results of the skin test and PCR were evaluated before and after ITAE, as well as the efficacy of ITAE according to patient and professional criteria. 152 patients were female and 174 were male for 46.6% and 53.4% respectively; those with 5 to 6 mm of haemorrhage were the most represented (p=0.04). There was a decrease in OSA severity levels after ITAE (p=0.025). In the assessment of the efficacy of ITAE, there was a significant number of improvements (p=0.012). PCR provides the diagnosis of OSA in AR, and ITAE changes the course of both conditions.

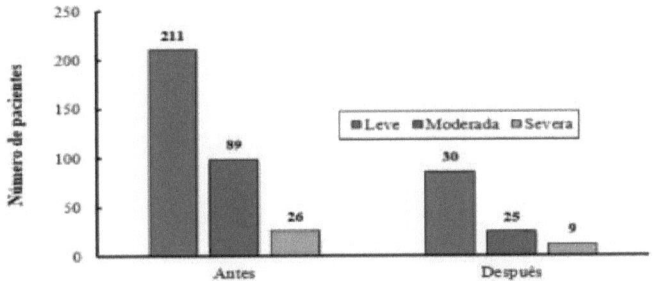

Niveles de gravedad antes y después de la ITAE

Another piece of equipment that can be used to diagnose SAHS is the PoKograph.
cardiorespiratory Sleep&Go (Fig. 4-4)

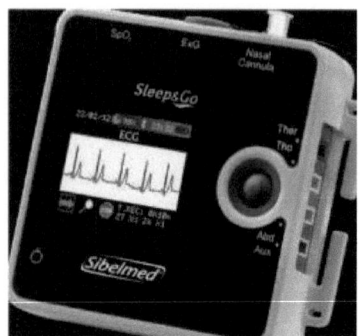

Fig. 4-4. Cardiorespiratory polygraph.
For the acquisition, storage and representation of biomedical signals necessary for a simplified diagnosis of SAHS, being any one or a combination of the following signals: respiratory flow, snoring, CPAP pressure measurement, thoracic effort, abdominal effort, oxygen saturation, beats per minute, plethysmographic waveform, limb movement, body position, activity and EEG-EMG-ECG signals.
Taken from the Sibelmed User Manual
Revision: 534-7AB-MU1 Rev. 1.10& 2017

The Sleep&Go has been designed for use by a physician or a trained technician for the acquisition of cardiorespiratory signals and the transmission of these signals to a PC during polygraphic studies.

The minimum age of the patient is 5 years old, with a weight over 15 kg and a minimum height of 70 cm. The medical staff will show the patient how to perform the test correctly, how to avoid interferences and how to place the sensors in their correct location in case they move.

The intended environments are hospitals, medical centers and sleep clinics. Studies can also be performed at the patient's home, with the exception of ExG signals (EEG, EOG, EMG, ECG).

While the Sleep&Go is recording, it is not allowed to use mobile phones, transmitters and similar equipment that generate radio frequency emissions near the system.

Treatment

The first thing in the treatment is to follow the ARIA evidence as detailed above for AR, keeping in mind that the treatments are very varied and depend on the cause of the apnea. In the case of patients with obesity, diet and exercise are basic. One of the options available is the implementation of a weight loss plan in the case of obstructive apnea, along with the avoidance of airway irritants. Treatment can be carried out in a variety of ways depending on the patient's needs and abilities, as well as their personal characteristics. In the American Journal of Respiratory and Critical Care Medicine, it is stated that weight loss is an effective treatment for apnea, but it is not yet known exactly why it produces this effect. It has been found that improvements in symptoms appear to be related to the reduction of fat on the tongue. Using MRI to measure the effect of weight loss on the upper airway in obese patients, researchers found that reducing tongue fat is a primary factor in reducing the severity of the disorder.

In a study it has been shown that a reduction in the volume of fat on the tongue is the main link between weight loss and improvement of sleep apnea. It was also found that weight loss resulted in a reduction of the pterygoid (jaw muscle that controls chewing) and lateral pharyngeal wall (muscles on the sides of the airways) volumes. Both of these changes also improved the sleep disorder, but not to the same extent as the reduction of tongue fat. There are treatment techniques, such as surgical tongue reduction.

Various drugs can be used in the treatment, although they are not always very effective. The exception may be if we are dealing with a patient whose obstruction is allergic or derived from different diseases expressed punctually. In these cases, the disease or disorder that causes or facilitates the disturbance of breathing during sleep should be treated, as we saw in AR with ITAE.

In some cases surgical intervention is required, for example when there is hypertrophy of the tonsils or even the tongue. Alternatives such as the use of dental prostheses or mandibular advancement devices can also be used.

If the mandible is small and backward, use mandibular advancement devices, which are placed in the mouth and solve the problem.

Internationally the three most common treatments of sleep apnea are:

- Continuous Positive Airway Pressure (CPAP). CPAP is the most common option and is the gold standard treatment.
- Automatic Positive Airway Pressure (APAP). This sleep apnea treatment automatically varies air pressure during the night to respond to changes in sleep.
- Bi-level treatment. This option is often used when a higher pressure is needed for effective sleep apnea treatment.

CPAP, or positive airway pressure treatment, uses a mask that delivers air at a slightly higher pressure than the ambient air pressure. The greatest achievements have been made in these devices that are small, portable and make little noise. It is a continuous positive airway pressure or CPAP mechanism that provides continuous pressure through a mask placed in the nose and/or mouth, allowing continued lung function by keeping the airways open. It is applied in those patients in whom nocturnal breathing problems are very frequent and do not respond to sleep hygiene and other treatments, and aims to achieve the cessation of apneas and respiratory flow limitation. Also the masks have been improved and are being tested some that are placed only in the nose and have improved the pipes that make the air to the nose.

Bibliography

Baharudin Abdullah, Kornkiat Snidvongs, Marysia Recto, Niken Lestari Poerbonegoro, De Yun Wang. Primary care management of rhinitis. Allergy: a cross-sectional study in four ASEAN countries. Multidisciplinary Respir Med. 2020 Dec 11; 15(1):726 doi: 10.4081/mrm.2020.726

Brozek et al. Allergic Rhinitis and its Impact on Asthma (ARIA) guidelines-2016 revision. J Allergy Clin Immunol 2017 Volume 140, Number 4:950-958

Nazar, G. (2013). Respiratory sleep disorders in the pediatric age. Revista Medica Clmica Las Condes, 24: 403-411. Elsevier.

Puertas FJ, Pin G, Santa Maria J, Duran Cantolla J. National Consensus on Sleep Apnea-Hypopnea Sleep Apnea Syndrome (SAHS). Spanish Sleep Group. Arch Bronchopneumol 2005: 41 (Suppl 4): 3-110.

Rodriguez Santos O, Garcia-Asensi A, Ponce Alvarez C, Galeana Rios R, Jardines Arciniega G, del Valle Monteagudo N. Importance of house mite allergens in the diagnosis of allergic rhinitis with sleep apnea hypopnea syndrome. Vaccimonitor 2019: 28 (3):97-102 www.vaccimonitor.finlay.edu.cu

Rodriguez Santos O, Garcia-Asensi A, del Valle Monteagudo N, Galeana Rios R, Flores Silveiro Z. Immunotherapy with mite allergens in patients with allergic rhinitis and obstructive sleep apnea. Vaccimonitor 2020: 29 (3):103-108 www.vaccimonitor.finlay.edu.cu

Sleep apnea treatment. Available at: www.resmed.com/es-xl/consumer/diagnosis-and-treatment/sleep-apnea/sleep-apnea-treatment/sleep- a...

Sleep disorders associated with medical and psychiatric illnesses (Esteban, Zamorano and Goncalvez, 2005. P, 30 - 31).

Chapter 5
Asthma and infection.

Dr. Edilberto Machado del Risco

Asthma and viral infection.

There is little doubt that there is a strong association between viral infections and the induction of wheezing illness and asthmatic exacerbations. The underlying mechanisms, although not precisely known, are probably multifactorial and involve inflammation of the bronchial mucosa, which interacts under certain circumstances with allergic inflammation. In addition, repeated infections play an important role in the perpetuation of inflammation and airway hyperresponsiveness (AVH), especially in the presence of atopy, a phenomenon that results in the transition from childhood asthma to a more persistent asthma phenotype.

The respiratory tract and immune system mature rapidly during the first years of life and postnatal lung development is affected and, in turn, influences responses to viral infections. Several factors, including age, type of virus, severity, location and timing of infection, in combination with the interaction of allergy and environmental contamination, have been implicated in the susceptibility of the lower airways to the effects of common respiratory viruses.

During the first two years of life children suffer from "immunological immaturity", because, although the human being is born with a repertoire of immune system cells capable of responding to any harmful stimulus, it takes time to generate responses, amplify the immune response and coordinate it in such a way that it is able to protect him/her. This immaturity is also conditioned by several factors, in chronological order in life: first of all, many more children are born by caesarean section and lose the opportunity of colonization by bacteria of vaginal bacterial flora, there are also many premature births, which conditions a lower transplacental passage of maternal immunoglobulin G (IgG), important to protect the young infant, and also a lack of exclusive breastfeeding for a long time in most of the cases.

In addition, it is important to consider that gastroesophageal reflux disease can affect up to 15-20% of infants in the first year of life; as the upper airways become irritated, milk regurgitates and gastric acid promotes epithelial damage that makes the infant more vulnerable to viral infection.

Respiratory viruses as inducers of asthma.

Bronchiolitis vinca is a common antecedent in children who later develop wheezing and asthma during childhood. The term bronchiolitis has been used since 1940 but has different meanings, as there is no unanimous consensus on its definition.

"Acute bronchiolitis refers to inflammation and obstruction of the lower respiratory tract, especially the small airways such as the bronchioles, causing distal air trapping accompanied by mild, moderate or severe respiratory distress. It is mostly caused by respiratory syncytial virus (RSV) infection, especially in children <2 years old.

In the last decade an increase in the incidence of hospitalizations for bronchiolitis is being described, where patients with bronchial hyperreactivity, family history of asthma and allergy, are more predisposed. Bronchiolitis is a self-limited disease, with low mortality in Cuba. It is clearly epidemic between September and March, although there may be sporadic cases throughout the year. The maximum peak is generally described in January or February; and it affects 10% of infants during an epidemic, of which 15 to 20% of the cases will require hospital admission.

There is much evidence linking early viral respiratory infections with the later development of asthma, but it is not yet sufficiently clear whether severe bronchiolitis is actually a cause of asthma or whether it is a susceptibility marker that signals children with a greater predisposition to develop asthma.

In studies in which all patients with a history of bronchiolitis have been analysed globally regardless of the causative virus, the prevalence of recurrent wheezing is 75% in the first two years of life, 47-59% at 2-4 years and 25-43% at 4-6 years, showing a clear decrease in the frequency of wheezing with age. However, long-term prospective follow-up studies of children hospitalized for bronchiolitis without considering the causative virus have shown a prevalence of asthma at 17-20 years of 41-43% in patients with a history of bronchiolitis compared to 11-15% in controls, and 35% at 25-30 years, with a significant impact on health-related quality of life.

These data indicate that not only is recurrent wheezing common in children after an episode of bronchiolitis, but also the recurrence of respiratory symptoms in young adults after a long asymptomatic period during school age and adolescence is frequent. This changes the previous concept of the relatively good prognosis of early childhood wheezing, demonstrating that the risk of asthma and impaired lung function may persist into adulthood.

Wittig and Glaser describe the existence of an epidemiological association between vmic bronchiolitis in infancy and the subsequent development of recurrent wheezing and/or asthma. Numerous studies have been published that have evaluated this relationship, although the different methodologies employed have made it difficult to draw conclusions that would unequivocally demonstrate this association. Nevertheless, in recent years several now classic prospective studies have shown that a history of RSV bronchiolitis is an independent risk factor for the development of recurrent wheezing and physician-diagnosed asthma.

The study by Sigurs et al., performed a longer follow-up of the cases that presented bronchiolitis in infancy, reaching 18 years of age at the last cut-off. The study included 47 infants under one year of age with severe bronchiolitis (hospitalized) due to RSV and 93 controls matched for age and sex. Children admitted for bronchiolitis had a higher prevalence of recurrent asthma/wheezing and allergic sensitization at 3, 7 and 13 years compared to the control group. At 18 years, the bronchiolitis group had a significantly higher prevalence of asthma (39% vs 9%), allergic rhinoconjunctivitis (43% vs 17%) and sensitization to perennial allergens (41% vs 14%). In addition, patients with a history of bronchiolitis had worse lung function (FEV1, FEV1/FVC) at 18 years of age than the control group, regardless of whether or not they had current asthma. Bronchial hyperresponsiveness and bronchodilator response were also more frequent in them. Finally, the only two risk factors independently related to the diagnosis of asthma at 18 years of age in this study were severe RSV bronchiolitis and the presence of allergic rhinoconjunctivitis. These results show that severe RSV bronchiolitis in the first months of life is associated with the development of asthma, bronchial hyperresponsiveness and allergic sensitization, and suggest that this association is maintained into adulthood.

Although RSV is undoubtedly the most frequent virus in the etiology of acute bronchiolitis in infants, the development of molecular diagnostic techniques, mainly polymerase chain reaction (PCR), has allowed us to know that other respiratory viruses, such as rhinoviruses, are also associated with bronchiolitis and probably with the development of asthma.

In Cuba there are reports that the months with the highest number of hospitalizations due to asthma are January, October, November and December, months with high viral circulation that imply these microorganisms as the cause of exacerbation crisis in cases with previous diagnosis of the disease, with higher presence in children under three years old and in males.

Asthma and bacterial infection.

It is very important the role played by the common or normal bacterial flora of the human respiratory tract, also the human nasopharynx is a natural reservoir of potentially pathogenic bacteria (BPP), which are involved in various infectious processes, especially in the infant population.

Among the main PPPs that cause respiratory infection are: *Staphylococcus aureus*, *Haemophilus influenzae*, *Moraxella catarrhalis*, *Streptococcus pneumoniae* and *Streptococcus pyogenes*. These bacteria colonize the nasopharynx of healthy individuals and contribute to the development of local or invasive infections. Their presence in the nasopharynx gives rise to the state of healthy carrier, a person who harbours an infectious agent without presenting clinical signs or symptoms of disease and who may constitute a potential source of infection and have been related to the perpetuation of the asthmatic process.

The risk factors that favor nasopharyngeal colonization by PPBs and the state of the carrier are several and among them are described: age, sex, smoking, passive smoking, lack of breastfeeding, alcohol consumption, overcrowding, occupation, acute respiratory infections (ARI), treatment with steroids, antimicrobials or immunosuppressive drugs, as well as allergic history (bronchial asthma), among others.

It is proposed that bacteria have the ability to secrete toxins, many of which can act as superantigens and under these conditions can modulate IgE synthesis. There are several examples such as *Staphylococcus aureus* which is able to stimulate inflammatory processes by excessive activation of T cells and macrophages, evidence of a new mechanism of immune stimulation in interaction with antigen presenting cells through MHC class II.

It has been described that some bacterial toxins can stimulate the activation of large numbers of TCD4+ lymphocytes and any of these toxins can stimulate all T cells in individuals expressing a particular "set" of T cell receptor-related genes. Such toxins are considered superantigens and their importance lies in their ability to stimulate effector mechanisms of the adaptive immune response with the subsequent appearance of clinicopathological abnormalities. Some T cells have receptors consisting of alpha and beta chains, which can stimulate, proliferate and secrete cytokines in response to superantigens.

Repeated acute respiratory infections of bacterial type appear in a significant group of asthmatics, a sustained exposure that makes the individual prone to the process of sensitization to the bacterial components. Once the individual has been sensitized, upon exposure to the originating anUgen or to another with similar characteristics, a series of immune mechanisms occur that give rise to the allergic response.

It is clear that bronchial asthma is a multifactorial disease whose decompensation is influenced by several causes, including living conditions, exposure to allergens and respiratory irritants, infections in early life, environmental pollution and its consequences. The correct diagnosis of which allergens sensitized the patient allows the proper management of the disease, avoiding contact and desensitizing therapy.

In Cuba, work is being done in this sense and efforts are being made to obtain bacterial extracts for allergological use, an aspect for which scientific evidence has been found. The use of desensitizing bacterial vaccines in the treatment of specific bacterial allergic sensitization is recognized by the allergological guild, but for its confection a standardization process is required to guarantee the immunogenicity of the product, stability, reproducibility and good clinical response; opportunity that is in the Center of Immunology and Biological Products (Cenipbi) of the Medical University of Camaguey, scientific center that develops research projects dedicated to the elaboration of vaccines destined to the allergy services.

The immunotherapy with therapeutic vaccines of bacterial lysate have proved to be effective in asthma with infectious component and in the asthma/EPOC phenotype, as shown by investigations developed in the allergy department of the hospital "Amalia Simoni" in Camaguey.

Asthma and intestinal parasitism.

The association between intestinal parasitosis and allergic diseases has not been fully established and remains contradictory; on the one hand, they have been linked as protective factors to the development of allergic diseases and on the other hand it is suggested that high parasite burden is a risk factor and contributes to the high prevalence of asthma and other allergic diseases in childhood. This relationship has also been studied for protozoa such as *Giardia lamblia*.

The interaction between helminths and atopy is conditioned by multiple factors, among which we can mention the time and duration of the first infection, the intensity of the infection, the genetic factors of the host and the type of parasite.

Helminths possess anUgens that stimulate an allergic inflammatory response by the host, which is associated with elevated IgE and cytokine production, predominantly IL-4, IL-5 and IL-13, characterizing a Th2 immune response, which generates an inflammatory response with a high eosinophilic load.

A study of 1004 children found that 260 were infected with A. lumbricoides and 233 had asthma. Parasite load was directly related to recurrent wheezing episodes. In children with higher parasite load, the presence of wheezing was much higher (p = 0.003, OR = 0.41, 95 CI 0.22 to 0.75), suggesting that this high parasite load is a risk factor contributing to the high prevalence of asthma and its symptoms.

Not only helminths have been studied to establish their relationship with allergy, but also protozoa. A study in children living in an urban area found the presence of *Giardia lamblia* in 45% of them, however, this was not related neither to allergic symptoms nor to skin tests.

Ibrahim Kassisse et al, studying the prevalence of allergic diseases in parasitized children did not find statistical significance ($x2$ = 2.30 < 3.84(1; 0.005), p = 1.29) between skin test positivity and parasitosis, but it is noteworthy that more than half of the children with positive prick were not parasitized. However, although no significant differences were found, the risk of skin test positivity was analyzed in relation to the type of parasite most frequently found. Children with Giardia lamblia infections had a risk of almost double when compared to those infected with Ascaris lumbricoides (OR = 1.14, CI 95: 0.36

to 3.62, p = 0.813 vs. OR = 0.16, CI 95: 0.02 to 1.36, p = 0.058).

Bibliography.

Backman K, Piippo-Savolainen E, Ollikainen H, Koskela H, Korppi M. Increased asthma risk and impaired quality of life after bronchiolitis or pneumonia in infancy. Pediatr Pulmonol. 2014[cited 2020 Oct 30]; 49:318-325. Available from: https://pubmed.ncbi.nlm.nih.gov/23836681/

Bragagnoli G, Silva MT. Ascaris lumbricoides infection and parasite load are associated with asthma in children. J Infect Dev Ctries. 2014; 8:891-7.

Camejo-Serrano Y, Morales-Torres G, EKas-Gonzalez J, Guerra-Dommguez E, Rivera-Morell M. Risk factors associated with bronchiolitis in children under two years of age. Bayamo. 2017-2019. MULTIMED [journal on the Internet]. 2020 [cited 2020 Oct 30]; 24(0): [approx. 10p .]. Available from:
http://www.revmultimed.sld.cu/index.php/mtm/article/view/1848

Campell DE, Kemp AS. Proliferation and production of interferon gamma and IL 4 in response to staphylococcal superantigen and staphylococcus aureus in chilhood atopic dermatitis. Clin. Exp Immunol 1997; 107(2): 392-97.

Cooper PJ, Barreto M, Rodrigues LC. Human allergy and geohelminth infections: a review of the literature and a proposed conceptual model to guide the investigation of possible causal associations. Br Med Bull. 2006; 79-80:203-18.

Cotrina Rico Karen Fiorella, Piedra Hidalgo Maria Fernanda, Chang Davila Domingo, Vega Vidal Marino, Osada Liy Jorge. Control of bronchial asthma in children and adolescents treated in health facilities in Chiclayo. Rev Cubana Pediatr [Internet]. 2020 Jun [cited 2020 Oct 30]; 92(2): e834. Available from: http://scielo.sld.cu/scielo.php?script=sciarttext&pid=S00347531202000020000 7&l ng=en.

Diego Rodriguez A, Dommguez Cortina G, Cubilla Tejeda A, Galindo Mendoza M. Acute respiratory infections, potential pathogenic bacteria, risk factors. Revista Salud Publica y Nutricion [Internet]. 2019[cited 2020 Oct 30]; 18 (4). [ca. 10p .]. Available In:
https://www.permanyer.com/wpcontent/uploads/2020/07/5522AX191infeccion

es.p df#page=11

Garrta Garrta M, Calvo Rey C, Rosal Rabes T. Asthma and viruses in the child. Arch Bronchopneumol. 2016 May [cited 2020 Oct 30]; 52(5): 269-273. Available from: https://www.ncbi.nlm.nih.gov/pmc/articles/PMC7131251/#bib0375

Garrta F, De la Cruz R. Update on the etiopathogenesis of acute bronchiolitis. 16 deApril [Internet]. 2018 [cited 2020 Oct 30]; 57(268):125-134. Available from: https://www.medigraphic.com/pdfs/abril/abr-2018/abr18268j.pdf

Global Initiative for Asthma. Global Strategy for Asthma Management and Prevention, Global Initiative for Asthma [Internet]. Fontana: GINA; 2017 [[cited 2020 Oct 30]. Available from: http://www.ginasthma.org.

Gonzalez AT, Cabrera MC, Gonzalez A, Gonzalez L, Triana Y. Behavior of wheezing in children under five years old in Sancti Spmitus province. Rev Inform Cient [journal on the Internet]. 2018 [cited 2020 Oct 30]; 97(3):[approx. 8p]. Available from: http://scielo.sld.cu/pdf/ric/v97n3/1028-9933-ric-9_7-03-538.pdf.

Goksor E, Alm B, Amark M, Ekerljung L, Lundback B, Wennergren G. High risk of adult asthma following severe wheeze in early life. Pediatr Pulmonol. 2015[cited 2020 Oct 30]; 50:789-799. Available from: https://pubmed.ncbi.nlm.nih.gov/25137605/

Kassisse EII, Surga Felix J, Torres Bermudez J, Kassisse JE. Prevalence of allergic diseases in parasitized children. Negative report of causality. Rev Pediatr Aten Primaria [Internet]. 2020 [cited 2020 Oct 30]; 22:e111-e119. Available

in: http://archivos.pap.es/files/11162867pdf/WEB_001RPAP_1507Prevalenciaalergia.pdf

Machado del Risco M, Nicolau Pestana E, Monde Enrique M. Standardization of bacterial extracts for use in allergological services. Tecnosalud [Internet]. 2016[cited 2020 Oct 30]. [approx. 10 p.]. Available from: http://tecnosalud2016.sld.cu/index.php/tecnosalud/2016/paper/viewFile/85/42

Machado del Risco E, Romero Gonzalez A, Nicolau Pestana E. Cellular sensitivity to bacteria in patients diagnosed with atopic dermatitis. AMC

[Internet]. 2009 [cited 2020 Oct 30], 13 (2): [approx. 10 p.]. Available from: http://scieloprueba.sld.cu/scielo.php?script=sciarttext&pid=S10250255200900 020 0003&lng=en&nrm=iso.

McConochie K.M. What's in the name? Am J Dis Child. 1983; 173:11-13.

Mendoza JA. Risk factors associated with bronchial asthma Hospital Nacional Sergio Enrique Bernales 2019 [Internet]. Lima: San Marth de Porres University; 2019 [cited 2020 Oct 30]. Available from: https://1library.co/document/q5ml3pwy-factoresasociados-bronquial-hospital-nacional-sergio-enrique-bernales.html.

Monde Enrique C, Machado del Risco E, Nicolau Pestana E. Bacterial immunotherapy in asthmatic patients with an infective component. Tecnosalud [Internet]. 2016[cited 2020 Oct 30]. [approx. 10 p.]. Available from http://tecnosalud2016.sld.cu/index.php/tecnosalud/2016/paper/viewFile/105/52

Munoz F. Asthma: endotypes and phenotypes in the pediatric age. Rev Alerg Mex [journal on the Internet]. 2019 [cited 2020 Oct 30]; 66(3):[approx. 5p]. Available from: http://www.scielo.org.mx/scielo.php?pid=S244891902019000300361&script=scielo.php?pid=S244891902019000300361&script=sciar ttext

Naranjo Rodriguez SA, Garrta Menendez R, Naranjo Rodriguez L, Negret Hernandez M. Use of immunotherapy in patients with Staphylococcus aureus infection. Rev med electron [Internet] 2011 [cited 2020 Oct 30]; 33(2): [approx. 10p .]. Available from URL: http://www.revmatanzas.sld.cu/revista%20medica/ano%202011/vol2%202011/tem a10.htm.

O'Callaghan-Gordo C., Bassat Q., D^ez-Padrisa N., Morais L., Machevo S., Nhampossa T. Lower respiratory tract infections associated with rhinovirus during infancy and increased risk of wheezing during childhood. A cohort study. PLoS One. 2013[cited 2020 Oct 30]; 8:e69370. Available from: https://pubmed.ncbi.nlm.nih.gov/23935997/

Paz Alvarez LA, Peralta Campos Y, Casado D^az S, Figueroa Perez E, Perez Alvarez OL . Management of acute bronchiolitis in the pediatric pneumology service of Pinar del Rfo. Rev. Medical Sciences [Internet]. 2020 [cited 2020

Oct30]; 24(5): e4460 .
in:
http://revcmpinar.sld.cu/index.php/publicaciones/article/view/4460

Sigurs N., Aljassim F., Kjellman B., Robinson P.D., Sigurbergsson F., Bjarnason R. Asthma and allergy patterns over 18 years after severe RSV bronchiolitis in the first year of life. Thorax. 2010 [cited 2020 Oct 30]; 65:1045-1052. Available from: https://pubmed.ncbi.nlm.nih.gov/20581410/

Stein M, Greenberg Z, Boaz M, Handzel ZT, Meshesha MK, Bentwich Z. The role of helminth infection and environment in the development of allergy: a prospective study of newly-arrived ethiopian immigrants in Israel. PLoS Negl Trop Dis. 2016; 10:e0004208.

Wammes LJ, Mpairwe H, Elliott AM, Yazdanbakhsh M. Helminth therapy or elimination: epidemiological, immunological, and clinical considerations. Lancet Infect Dis. 2014; pii: S1473-3099.

Wammes LJ, Mpairwe H, Elliott AM, Yazdanbakhsh M. Helminth therapy or elimination: epidemiological, immunological, and clinical considerations. Lancet Infect Dis. 2014; pii: S1473-3099.

Webb EL, Nampijja M, Kaweesa J, Kizindo R, Namutebi M, Nakazibwe E, et al. Helminths are positively associated with atopy and wheeze in Ugandan fishing communities: results from a cross-sectional survey. Allergy. 2016; 71:1156-69.

Wittig H.J., Glaser J. The relationship between bronchiolitis and childhood asthma: A follow-up study of 100 cases of bronchiolitis. J Allergy. 1959 [cited 2020 Oct 30]; 30:19-23. Available from: https://pubmed.ncbi.nlm.nih.gov/13620441/

Yanes-Martas J, D^az-Ceballos J, Fonseca-Hernandez M, Garrta-Rodriguez I, Llul-Tombo C, Tio-Gonzalez D. Clinical, epidemiological and therapeutic characteristics of patients admitted for bronchial asthma crisis. Revista Finlay [journal on the Internet]. 2020 [cited 2020 Oct 30]; 10(3): [approx. 8 p.]. Available from: http://revfinlay.sld.cu/index.php/finlay/article/view/789

Yasuda K, Nakanishi K. Host responses to intestinal nematodes. Int Immunol. 2018; 30:93-102.

Chapter 6
Asthma in the life-threatening child
Author: Dr.C Valentin Santiago Rodriguez Moya

It is evident that the ability to breathe is a determining and characteristic function of all living beings. Whenever any of the physiological processes associated with breathing fail, life is compromised. Breathing, however, goes beyond the movement of air in the lung structures, it involves the possibility of refreshing the air in the alveoli so that the exchange of gases occurs with the blood according to the needs of the different organs and systems, and is called external respiration. However, chemists, biochemists, and physiologists are familiar with a more subtle step in the respiratory processes, namely the use and production of the gases handled by the lungs during vital metabolic activity, and this is called internal respiration. The external respiratory phenomena must be coupled to the demands of internal respiration.

The care of the paediatric population in the emergency department begins with the paediatric assessment triangle (PET), continues with the ABCDEF to stabilize the patient, where the (F) that refers to the family must be well explained to avoid misinterpretation in the critically ill patient and ends with the history taking and exploration to try to reach a diagnosis. The application of the PET scan consists of a rapid assessment (30-60 seconds) of the general appearance (appearance), respiratory effort and skin colour (circulation), which constitute the three edges of the triangle. The main pathophysiological diagnoses that can be established depend on the altered sides of the triangle: stable, central nervous system dysfunction, respiratory distress, respiratory failure, circulatory failure or *shock*, decompensated *shock* and cardiopulmonary failure. Children with altered level of consciousness represent a diagnostic and therapeutic challenge. Organized care using the PET scan and ABCDEF will allow assessment of the severity of the condition and management according to symptomatology. It is important to recognize the clinical signs of risk of permanent brain damage or death to avoid delays and to make a broad differential diagnosis to establish a definitive treatment in those cases that require it.

Asthma is a syndrome that includes several clinical phenotypes that share similar clinical manifestations, but have different causes. It is defined as a chronic inflammatory disease of the airways, involving different cells and inflammatory mediators, conditioned in part by genetic factors, which presents with bronchial hyperresponsiveness and a variable obstruction to total or reversible airflow, either by drug action or spontaneously. Being a chronic disease, the objective of its approach is to maintain control of it and the prevention of serious complications, which can endanger the life of the pediatric patient and generate an emotional crisis to the family.

It is estimated that more than half of adults with asthma were already asthma in childhood, hence the importance of identifying it early in life, during the first 1000 days (2 years), the definition, diagnostic criteria and even the classification of asthma are complicated and subject to controversy, This is because the usual symptoms (coughing, wheezing and shortness of breath) are common in children under 3 years of age without asthma and also because of the impossibility of routinely evaluating lung function. Definitive diagnosis requires exclusion of other diseases that may present with similar signs and symptoms. In reference to the characteristics of the child population, tools or models have been developed to predict the future risk of asthma, but few have been validated. The best known is the Predictive Asthma Index (PAI), established from the study of the Tucson cohort, so far is the most useful, being simple to perform, the best validated and have a better positive likelihood ratio. The diagnosis of asthma in children under 3 years of age must be probable, and this probability is increased if atopy is present. The term asthma should not be avoided when there are more than 3 episodes per year, or severe episodes, of cough, wheezing and shortness of breath, with good response to maintenance treatment with inhaled corticosteroids and if there is a worsening after their withdrawal.

1. Pathophysiology of severe asthma

Local cellular events in the airway have important effects on lung function. As a consequence of airway inflammation with edema and mucus hypersecretion and muscle hyperreactivity, airway obstruction occurs. The consequent reduction of the airway lumen with obstruction to airflow leads to:

— Increased flow resistance, predominantly expiratory.

— Air trapping by dynamic hyperinflation, with positive self-pressure at the end of exhalation.

— Heterogeneity of pulmonary gas distribution with alterations of the ventilation/perfusion ratio.

Exhalation allows emptying of the alveoli with return to the resting volume of the respiratory system at the end of expiration. Airflow obstruction during expiration is manifested by a decrease in forced expiratory volume in the first second, forced expiratory volume in the first second/forced vital capacity ratio, mesoexpiratory flow and maximal expiratory flow. These changes are accompanied by

a decrease in vital capacity, an increase in residual volume and functional residual capacity, contributes to dynamic hyperinflation and air trapping.

Dynamic hyperinflation can be defined as the failure of the lung volume to reach the end-expiratory relaxation volume before the beginning of the next inhalation, which is the cause of a positive pressure in the alveoli at the end of the exhalation (positive end-expiratory intrinsic pressure or positive end-expiratory self-pressure), which conditions an increase in the elastic respiratory work and contributes to respiratory muscle fatigue.

Although the pulmonary distension caused by dynamic hyperinflation can generate certain beneficial effects (maintenance of airway patency with decreased resistance and better distribution of ventilation), the adverse effects on hemodynamics and pulmonary mechanics on the patient are predominant:

— Increased elastic work.
— Increased inspiratory threshold load (in assisted and spontaneous ventilation). - Increased oxygen consumption.
— Diaphragmatic flattening, with compromise of the respiratory pump.
— Increased dead space.
— Fast and shallow breathing.
— Asynchroma patient/respirator.
— Respiratory acidosis.
— Drop in venous return and cardiac minute volume, arterial hypotension. - Airway block.

The respiratory rate is elevated during an acute asthmatic crisis. This tachypnoea is not caused by alterations in arterial gas composition, but by stimulation of intrapulmonary receptors, with consequent effects on the central respiratory centres. A consequence of the combination of airway narrowing and rapid flows is an increased mechanical load on the ventilatory pump and in severe asthma the ventilatory load or workload may increase and predispose to ventilatory muscle fatigue and consequent respiratory failure.

The predominant pathophysiological mechanism leading to hypoxemia is the alteration of the ventilation/perfusion ratio, due to the irregular distribution of ventilation. The sectorial nature of the narrowing of the airway causes a poor distribution of ventilation (V) in relation to irrigation (Q), that is, ventilation/perfusion ratio (V/Q) less than 1, its net effect is the cause of arterial hypoxemia, arterial hypocapnia due to hyperventilation and altered alveolar arterial oxygen difference (PAO2 - PaO2). Hypoxemia is correctable with inspired oxygen fraction of 28% to 40% in most episodes. In cases of greater severity and duration such as the one that occupies us this chapter, can be observed accentuation of hypoxemia and hypercapnia and metabolic acidosis. Respiratory acidosis is the result of increased dead space due to alveolar overdistension, accentuation of ventilation/perfusion disorders and inability of the muscular pump to maintain sufficient alveolar ventilation in the face of the increased work of breathing that it has to cope with.

2. Clfnical gravity:

Severe acute asthma describes a severe asthma attack that puts the patient at risk of developing respiratory failure, a condition formerly known as *status asthmaticus* or *status asthmaticus*. The time course of the attack as well as the severity of the airway obstruction can vary over the course of the condition. The classification of severity is different according to the moment at which it is made: at the beginning, at the time of diagnosis or later, once control has been achieved. In the first case, the level of severity depends on the frequency and intensity of symptoms (number of crises and the situation between them, exercise tolerance and nocturnal symptoms), the need for rescue bronchodilators and the values of the functional respiratory examination. In young children in whom it is not possible to perform a pulmonary function study, severity is classified according to symptomatology.

The following should be considered: the time of evolution of the crisis, the pharmacological treatment administered, the existence of associated diseases and possible risk factors (previous intubation or admission to care units for the critically ill patient, hospitalization in the previous year, use of oral glucocorticoids, excessive use of short-acting beta agonists (SABA) in the previous weeks).

The assessment of severity is based on clinical criteria (respiratory rate, presence of wheezing and the existence of sternocleidomastoid muscle retractions). Although no clinical scale is well validated, the *Pulmonary Score (Table 1)* is simple and applicable to all ages. The symptoms, together with transcutaneous oxygen saturation by pulse oximetry (SpO2), complete the estimation of the severity of the episode.

Table 1. Pulmonary Score

Pulmonary Score for the clinical assessment of asthma attacks in children*.				
Score	FR**		Wheezing	Use of sternocleidomastoid
	<6 years	> 6 years		
0	< 30	< 20	No	No
1	31-45	21-35	End exhalation	Slight increase
2	46-60	36-50	Whole exhalation (stethoscope)	Enhanced

Respiratory rate
If there is no wheezing and the sternocleidomastoid activity is increased, score

	> 60	> 50	Maximum activity
3		Breathing in and out without stethoscope***.	

It is scored 0 to 3 in each of the sections (minimum 0, maximum 9). the wheezing section with a 3.

During the global assessment of the severity of asthma exacerbation in children, integration of the above results with SpO2 is used (Table 2).

Table 2. Global assessment of the severity of asthma exacerbation in children.

SpO2*. In case of discordance between the clinical score and the oxygen saturation, the most severe will be used. It is considered severe with a score

Pulmonary Score and oxygen saturation are integrated.		
	Pulmonary Score	SpO2* SpO2* SpO2* SpO2* SpO2* SpO2* SpO2
Slightly	0-3	> 94 %
Moderate	4-6	91-94 %
Serious	7-9	< 91 %

from the concept of moderate.

3. Laboratory and radiological findings

Numerous studies are necessary and may be useful to accurately assess the extent of severity, response to treatment, presence of complications and alternative diagnoses, but in critically ill patients they should not precede or condition initial treatment.

3.1 - Hemogasometry

The hemogasometric study is essential to evaluate the alterations in the gaseous exchange that includes uptake, transport and cession of oxygen and also provides the basic information to evaluate the response to the imposed therapy, orients in the direction of the decrease of the arterial oxygen pressure, the oxygen saturation and also, in the sense of determining the adequate efficiency of the pulmonary ventilation according to the level of arterial pressure of carbon dioxide.

Other aspects that can be determined through arterial hemogasometry is the acid-base and electrolyte status of the patient. In the early stages there is respiratory alkalosis, but if maintained for hours or days, a renal retention of bicarbonate may arise, which may be expressed late as a metabolic acidosis with normal GAP anion.

Respiratory acidosis may coexist with lactic acidosis and may be a common cause of elevated GAP anion, its pathogenesis in acute severe asthma is not yet elucidated and appears to be a consequence of several mechanisms:
— The use of high doses of beta-2-agonists.
— The manifest increase in the work of the respiratory muscles resulting in anaerobic metabolism and overproduction of lactic acid.
— The coexistence of profound tissue hypoxia.
— The presence of intracellular alkalosis.
— Decreased lactate clearance by the ^gado due to tissue hypoperfusion and some passive congestion of the ^gado due to the establishment of high intrathoracic pressures.

3.2 - Blood count

In the patient with catarrhal symptoms, fever, cough and respiratory distress or one of these situations, a complete blood count should be performed in order to document the presence of leukocytosis or deviation to the left to suspect bacterial processes as a precipitating factor, in addition to verifying the content of hemoglobin, among others. The leukocyte and lymphocyte count orients us about the immunological status and also allows us to take strategies after discharge.

3.3 - Electrolyte analysis

It is prudent to monitor electrolytes in patients with ascites, cardiovascular disease, diuretics and steroids because excessive use of beta agonists can decrease serum potassium levels in up to 70% of cases. Sodium should also be monitored, as severe asthma is associated with the syndrome of inadequate secretion of antidiuretic hormone, which can cause hyponatremia. Respiratory alkalosis is sometimes accompanied by over-added hypochloremia.

3.4 - Chest X-ray

The initial and evolutionary value of the chest X-ray is unquestionable and should never be forgotten. Often the chest X-ray of a patient with asthma is normal in the early stages or radiological changes are seen nonspecific to the disease. Sometimes chronic air trapping images are visualized and in young children we can visualize the size of the thymic gland and infer the number of respiratory infections it has undergone previously according to its size.

Severe asthma is associated with pulmonary hyperinflation manifested by lowering of the diaphragm and abnormal radiolucency of the lung fields, and pneumothorax, pneumomediastinum and atelectasis as a complication can be detected by this route. Radiological studies are useful in the evaluation of a new onset wheezing crisis, especially in the infant population.

Patients with no previous history of asthma should always have a chest X-ray to rule out congenital cardio vascular malformations with increased pulmonary flow. A poor response to treatment, the presence of fever, purulent sputum and leukocytosis is an indication for the study. Signs of pneumomediastinum, subcutaneous emphysema, and spontaneous pneumothorax make it necessary to perform the study urgently. Another usefulness is that it can contribute to the differential diagnosis of other causes of respiratory failure (foreign bodies, viral or aUpical pneumomas and cystic fibrosis).

3.5 - Other tests

Some are considered optional, such as glycemia (hyperglycemic effect of beta agonists and steroids), creatinine and urinary density (for undiscovered insensible loss of free water through the respiratory tract, fever and diuresis increased by aminophylline, diuretics, rule out the presence of diabetes ins^pidus, among others).

3.6 - Examination of bronchial secretions

The appearance of yellow, brownish or bloody sputum is suggestive of pneumoma and in these cases it is useful to indicate microbiological study of sputum that can be useful for the diagnosis of the existing germ. The culture of the sputum is an important procedure in cases where age allows it, otherwise those who are coupled to a mechanical respiration equipment, can be cultured secretions from the mouth and bronchial secretions as a method to guide the antimicrobial policy to follow.

In other cases, cytologic studies of the expectorated secretions may be indicated, which will orientate

to differentiate the presence of eosinophils (acute or chronic crisis due to allergic reactions) or neutrophils (presence of respiratory infection).

4. Hospitalization Criteria

One of the most difficult aspects for the intensivist, for the emergency physician or for the on-call physician is when to admit an asthmatic patient to the intensive care unit. Every asthmatic patient who presents a severe acute crisis and does not resolve with the usual therapy is tributary to admission to the intensive care unit, however, it requires a guideline to be assessed at the time of deciding to

admit an asthmatic to the intensive care unit: - Multiple visits to the emergency room.
— Failure of outpatient therapy.
— Asthmatic with a history of endotracheal intubation with admission to the intensive care unit, who does not have a rapid recovery after 1 h of treatment.
— Asthmatics with signs of physical exhaustion.
— Asthmatics with signs of inflammatory condensation or airway blockage.
— Pneumoma with hypoxemia.
— Need for oxygen therapy to achieve SpO2above 92%.
— Progressive loss of consciousness. A decrease in Glasgow scale (or modified Glasgow scale for minors) over a period of one hour.
— Polypnoea and tachycardia maintained despite initial treatment.
— Asthmatic with alterations in blood gases: respiratory acidosis with metabolic alkalosis.

5. Treatment

The education of the child with asthma and his family increases the quality of life and reduces the risk of exacerbations and health costs, so it is one of the cornerstones of treatment. Its aim is for the child to achieve a normal life for his or her age, including physical activity and sport.

The goal of initial therapeutic measures is to reverse bronchial obstruction and hypoxia as quickly as possible and to institute or revise the therapeutic plan to prevent further crises. All patients with severe respiratory distress should initially receive supplemental oxygen by the best tolerated and most appropriate method to achieve the required oxygen concentration and appropriate doses of nebulized beta-2-agonists should be administered. These measures can be summarized as follows:

— Maintenance of adequate arterial oxygen saturation with the administration of supplemental oxygen.
— Decrease airway obstruction and improve airflow limitation as soon as possible with fast-acting bronchodilators (beta agonists and anticholinergics).
— Restore lung function as soon as possible by improving airway inflammation through the use of corticosteroid by systemic route.
— Identify and treat the causal or triggering factor.
— Do not delay initiating intensive specific treatment.

5.1- <u>General measures</u>

5.1.1 - Prepare the reception in the Intensive Care Unit:
- Prepare conditions for the boarding of the airplane.
- Have a multimodal lung ventilator.

5.1.2 - Adequate position: to allow the patient to ventilate better (30o to 45o *fowler* position). In small children we must be very careful with the hyperextension of the neck.

5.1.3 - Oxygen therapy: All patients with severe asthma attacks have a variable degree of hypoxemia. Monitoring with a pulse oximeter of SpO2 and administration of supplemental oxygen should be the first actions at the beginning of the evaluation and medical treatment, with the objective of maintaining an SpO2 greater than 92% (greater than 95% in pregnant paediatric patients), taking into account that the priority is to neutralize tissue hypoxia, the essential mechanism of death.

Before administering inhaled salbutamol we must administer oxygen because several studies have shown hypoxemia if the drug is administered without prior oxygenation.

Oxygen should be administered humidified. The flow from 1 L/min to 4 L/min, using nasal catheter and nasal cannulas, it is advisable to use masks based on the Venturi principle, when there is hypercapnia, (some dyspneic patients may develop a feeling of claustrophobia), indicating increasing concentrations (24%, 28% and 31%) until the desired saturation is reached. So-called "high oxygen flows" (inspired oxygen fraction greater than 35%) are not recommended. Hyperoxia can be harmful and may be associated with hypercapnia. Demonstration of hypoxemia refractory to oxygen administration once treatment is initiated should suggest complications.

5.1.4 - Hydration: the calculation must be made in relation to the daily needs and according to the existence of an imbalance in the water metabolism.
- Less than 10 Kg: 100 ml/kg/ 24 hours.
- From 11-20 Kg weight: 1000 ml + 50 ml/kg/ 24 hours for each kg 'over 10.
- Over 20 kg: 1000 ml + 20 ml/kg for each kg over 20 kg.

It must be rational to maintain an adequate balance according to the need to replace losses due to tachypnea and fever in case of infection. During the replenishment of losses the following measures should be executed:
- Taking vital signs every 1 h.
- Cardiovascular monitoring and SpO2.

- Abundant liquid diet. If vomiting occurs or the patient is intubated, a nasogastric tube should be placed.
- Ensure permeable airway.
- Aspiration of airway secretions should be performed when there is evidence that they are present, but repeated unexplained aspiration should be avoided because it may induce bronchospasm.

5.1.5 - Humidification of the airway: the use of heated humidifiers is preferred, to avoid too high or too low temperatures, which can induce bronchospasm.

5.1.6 - Complementary examinations: thorax x-rays on admission, then daily; blood gases according to clinical status and ventilatory parameters; daily haemochemical and haematological tests.

5.1.7- Use of antibiotics: asthma precipitated by infection is caused by non-bacterial agents and bronchospasm is the result of airway inflammation and should be treated in the same way as other asthma attacks. The use of empine antibiotics is not justified. Antibiotic therapy in a patient with an asthma attack is only indicated if bacterial infection is present.

5.1.8 - Respiratory physiotherapy: in the first phase it is likely that active kinesiotherapy on the patient in crisis will only trigger more bronchial obstruction, so at this stage it is only indicated to use methods that relax the muscles. When the patient begins to experience improvement, diaphragmatic mobilization therapy, bronchial drainage and breathing exercises can be initiated.

5.1.9 - Identify and influence precipitating factors.

5.1.10 - Do not delay initiating intensive sperm treatment.

6. Drugs with primarily bronchodilator action

6.1- Beta-2-adrenergic agonists

In 1968 a team of researchers from Glaxo synthesized the first selective agonist for beta 2 adrenoreceptors called salbutamol, although its duration remained short and therefore called SABA (*Short Action Beta Agonist*) that until today has been used for the control of acute asthma attacks and the same Glaxo team progressively synthesized other bronchodilators with longer duration of action (salmeterol, formoterol and indacaterol) with action times between 12 h and 24 h, which were called long-acting beta agonists, LABA (*Long Action Beta Agonist*).

Among the SABA, the most widely used drug is salbutamol. They are the first line of treatment because of their greater effectiveness and fewer adverse reactions. In the treatment of acute asthma, they should be administered with a pressurized inhaler and spacer chamber, since this form of administration is as effective as that of nebulizers in the treatment of acute asthma. The recommended doses and administration times depend on the severity of the attack and the response to the initial doses. Nebulized SABA should be restricted only to cases where the patient requires oxygen to normalize SpO2, although a recent randomized clinical trial (RCT) showed that, even in severe attacks, salbutamol and ipratropium bromide with a spacer chamber and oxygen face mask administered via nasal cannula was more effective than by nebulizer. Continuous nebulization does not offer great advantages over intermittent nebulization at equal total doses administered. Table 3 shows the most commonly used inhaled beta-2 agonists.

Table 3. Characteristics of beta-2-agonists for inhalation use

Bronchodilator	Start of from action	Duration of action	Therapeutic use
SABA			
Salbutamol	<5 min	3-6 h	110-200 цд four times
Terbutaline	<5 min	4-6 h	500 цд four times a day
LABA			
Salmeterol	=15 min	12 h	50-100 ц twice a day
Vilanterol	=5 min	12 h	55 цд once a day
Formoterol	=10 min	12 h	>6 years 12mcg/12h not to exceed 24mcg/day
Ultra-LABA			
Indacaterol	=5 min	24 h	150-300 цд once daily

LABA are not widely used in clinical practice during acute bronchial asthma crises, which involve admission to intensive care, but very often ambulatory asthma patients receive them chronically associated with inhaled steroids, which is why it is important that the intensivist knows their main characteristics, because of the interactions they may have with the treatment of acute crises.

Other drugs mentioned are those that act by stimulating beta-1-adrenergic receptors, which cause an increase in heart rate, increased cardiac contractility and myocardial oxygen consumption; stimulation of beta-2-adrenergic receptors causes dilation of bronchial and vascular smooth muscle, tremor, decreased cellular inflammatory response. The adrenergic response causes vascular smooth muscle contraction with increased systemic resistances.

Epinephrine was the first beta-adrenergic agonist used in the treatment of asthma, but its undesirable alpha 1 and beta 1-adrenergic effects caused many controversies about its use and its routes of administration. Later, isoproterenol appeared with better bronchodilator activity and less alpha 1-adrenergic effect, that is, it is not a selective agonist of beta 2 receptors. Later, isohetarin appeared as a beta agonist with beta 2 activity and weak beta 1 activity, with short periods of action. Both drugs were used for a long time, but it was necessary to modify the structure of catecholamines to increase the selectivity for beta 2-adrenoreceptors, to reduce the disadvantages of their undesirable alpha 1 and beta 1-adrenergic effects and to achieve a higher bioavailability. Thus arose metaproterenol as the first selective beta-2 receptor agonist, followed by terbutaline and albuterol (salbutamol) and more recently a new generation of highly selective beta-2-agonists of longer action, formoterol, salmeterol and others, but their use is not accepted in acute access, given their slower onset of action and the longer duration of possible side effects.

For some years now, fast-acting beta-2-agonists have been the most effective bronchodilators available, the treatment of choice in asthma attacks. The mechanism of action of beta agonists has been well studied. In the lung, stimulation of beta-2 receptors promotes the activation of Gs stimulatory coupling protein, which stimulates the activation of the enzyme adenylyl cyclase, resulting in an increase in the rate of synthesis of cfclic adenosine monophosphate from adenosine triphosphate. This increase in cfclic adenosh monophosphate accelerates the inactivation of A-type kinases of myosin light chains and facilitates the expulsion of calcium from the cell or its sequestration in the sarcoplasmic muscle, leading to relaxation in smooth muscle.

Their action lies in smooth muscle relaxation, with the resulting bronchodilation, increase mucociliary transport, increase the activity of cilia and modify the composition of mucous secretions. They also provide other benefits, acting on endothelial cells and inflammatory cells, it is specified that:

— They decrease the release of histamine from both basophils and mast cells and of prostaglandin D2 by mast cells.

— They inhibit the oxidative burst and the release of thromboxane and C4 leukotrienes by eosinophils.

— Inhibit cytokine release by monocytes and lymphocytes.

— It favors the desensitization of the alveolar macrophages.

— They inhibit the oxidative function of neutrophils and the release of mediators.

Table 4. Beta-agonists and doses to be administered during crisis

Beta agonists	Inhalation vfa dose	Subcutaneous vfa dose	Intravenous vfa dose
Albuterol or salbutamol	Initial: 0.15 mg/kg per dose diluted in saline 0.9% 4ml, up to three doses every twenty minutes. Then every one to four hours if necessary. We can also double the indicated dosage regardless of any reactions adverse reactions. Continuous nebulization 0,5mg/kg/hour		Initial bolus of 10mcg/kg over 10 to 20 minutes, may be increased by 0.2mcg/kg/minute until 1mcg/kg/minute to improve bronchospasm or adverse reactions appear
Terbutaline 1mg=1ml	0.1mg/kg per dose diluted in 0.9% saline up to three doses not exceeding 0.3mg per administration	0.01mg/kg/dose 15-20 minutes up to three doses. Maximum dose 0,5mg/4h if necessary.	2-10 mcg/kg/load dose followed by infusion of 0.1 to 0.4mcg/kg/minute
Adrenaline 1mg=1ml		0.01mg/kg/dose (1:1000) 15 20 minutes up to three doses. Maximum dose 0,3mg	Continuous perfusion 0,01 Rg/kg/min to 0.15 g/kg/min
Levalbuterol/Levsalbutamol	0.075 mg/kg (minimum dose 1.25 mg) every 20 minutes for 3 doses, then 0.075- 0.15 mg/kg up to 5 mg every 1-4 hours as needed.		

6.1.2. Inhaled fast-acting beta-2-agonists

Albuterol (salbutamol) is the cornerstone of treatment of exacerbations in patients with acute asthma. It should be indicated in the severely ill asthmatic with an initial dose of 0.15 mg/kg/dose (0.5% solution) in 4 to 5 mL of 0.9% saline solution by nebulization every 20 min of three doses at a flow rate of 6 L/min to 8 L/min, it can be administered every 1 h to 4 h, as needed, spacing them more as improvement progresses. Continuous nebulization should be considered in the most severe patients. Tachycardia and hypokalemia may occur with continuous therapy.

Another alternative is the use of levalbuterol/Levsalbutamol, dose regulated by age, where 0.63 mg are equivalent to 1.25 mg of albuterol with the same efficacy and less adverse reactions. For continuous nebulization, 5 mg/h to 7.5 mg/h is recommended.

6.1.3. Subcutaneous therapy with beta-2-agonists

Epinephrine and terbutaline used subcutaneously are powerful tools in critical situations. Their administration should be considered in patients who do not respond to continuous nebulized salbutamol and in those unable to cooperate due to neurological depression. In addition, it can be used in ventilated patients who do not respond to inhalation therapy. Subcutaneous beta agonist therapy has a disadvantage in terms of therapeutic/toxicity ratio compared to selective inhaled beta-2 agonists. Although there is no proven value that the subcutaneous route provides better results over nebulized therapy, rapid administration of beta agonists to the airway may be of benefit in some asthmatic patients who are at imminent risk of respiratory failure and at low risk of cardiac toxicity such as children. In this circumstance, a combined administration of both routes may be useful.

Subcutaneous terbutaline is recommended in pregnancy because it appears to be safer than epinephrine. Adrenaline infusion has been used to treat severe crises of bronchial asthma, with recommendable results, especially in patients who are submitted to mechanical artificial ventilation, thus the taboos that it was not recommendable to use it when there was a severe respiratory acidosis have been unfounded, because it could induce severe cardiac arrhythmias, when in practice its use and the improvement of oxygenation reduce tachycardia and bronchospasm more efficiently, without inducing severe cardiac arrhythmias.

With parenteral administration, adrenaline has a rapid onset of action and a short duration of approximately 5 min, which is shorter if administered intravenously, is rapidly metabolized by the liver, kidney, skeletal muscle and mesenteric organs, and is degraded to an inactive metabolite called vanillylmandelic acid by enzymatic effects. The occurrence of tachycardia and hypertension should be monitored during infusion use, although these occur infrequently when use and dosage are appropriate.

1.2. Methylxanthines

Methylxanthine derivatives (aminophylline/theophylline) have been used for many years as first-line bronchodilator therapy in the treatment of asthma attacks, however, their poor therapeutic margin, the need to monitor plasma levels, the better efficiency of beta-2-agonist therapy and doubts regarding the association with inhaled beta-2-agonist adrenergics in the improvement of lung function have questioned their use.

As a single therapy it is less effective in patients with asthmatic crisis than other available therapies, in spite of what has been published in different studies, which do not show conclusive results, treatment with aminophylline is recommended in hospitalized patients. In Cuba its use continues and future research will shed more light and precision on this drug in hospitalized severe asthmatic patients, although there is enough consensus in using it when there is an incomplete or bad response to the combined use of beta-2-agonists, anticholinergics, steroids and in patients who need mechanical ventilatory support.

Aminophylline is the intravenous solution of theophylline, which contains approximately 80 % theophylline. The ampoule of aminophylline for parenteral use contains 200 mg. When theophylline enters the circulation, approximately 70 % is bound to plasma proteins and the remainder is distributed over the body surface with lower concentrations in adipose tissue; serum concentrations reach equilibrium with tissue concentrations of the drug 1 h after intravenous administration and 90% is metabolized in the liver by cytochrome P450 into inactive metabolites that are excreted in the urine, so that any impairment of hepatic function or renal clearance of theophylline increases its blood concentration and the risk of toxicity if standard doses are continued without monitoring of plasma levels.

The cellular mechanism by which theophylline exerts its actions is still not clear. Xanthines inhibit calcium adenosine monophosphate phosphodiesterase, increase the levels of these nucleotides and alter intracellular Ca^{2+} mobilization, leading to muscle relaxation and inhibition of the inflammatory response. Today it is known that the concentration of the drug necessary to increase the cAMP in vitro, exceeds the therapeutic levels in vivo. The most widely accepted hypothesis of action is based on the ability of xanthines to block A1 and A2 adenosine receptors at concentrations equivalent to therapeutic levels. Despite the current controversy over use, other factors have been proposed that may help explain the favorable effects of theophylline:

— Stimulates the release of endogenous catecholamines.
— It has certain anti-inflammatory actions.
— Inhibits the release of mediator substances by the mastocyst.
— Inhibits the formation of prostaglandins and antagonizes adenosine.
— Improves mucociliary clearance.
— Stimulates the ventilatory bellows.
— Increases diaphragmatic contractility and prevents diaphragmatic muscle fatigue.
— Increases diuresis.
— Decreases preload and afterload.

In practice, a loading dose of 5 mg/kg intravenous infusion in 20 min to 30 min is used in patients who have not received methylxanthine treatment, reaching concentrations of 10 pg/dL to 15 pg/dL. When the patient has received 6 h before intravenous aminophylline, a dose of 2.5 mg/kg in 20 min is safe and care should be taken that the attack dose does not exceed 6 mg/kg to 7 mg/kg when the previous and current doses are added together.

Then an age-dependent infusion is used. The infusion rate should be adjusted taking into account other clinical situations or drugs used that can synergistically alter the metabolism of xanthines, there are ranges of doses for administration in different clinical situations, which is expressed in Table 5.

Table 5. Use of aminophylline in the paediatric age group

Age	Aminophylline mg/kg/h
1-6 months	0,5
7-12 months	0,85
1-9 years	1
More than 9 years	0,75
Increases the metabolism of theophylline	Phenytoin(75%), Isoproterenol(15-20%), Barbiturates(25%)
Decrease the metabolism of theophylline	Alupurinol(25%), Propanolol(20%), Erythromycin/25%), Cimetidine(25-100%), oral contraceptives(35%).

If there are conditions to measure the serum levels of theophylline, it is recommended to perform this measurement 1 h after the attack doses and 6 to 8 h after starting the intravenous infusion and continue every day, as long as the infusion persists or the infusion dose can be reduced due to clinical and gasometric improvement; it should be remembered that concentrations higher than 20 pg/mL, constitute the toxic level of the drug and forces to reduce the dose, although sometimes begin to see toxic manifestations between 15 pg/mL to 20 pg/mL, ie, very close to therapeutic levels, so that whenever this drug is used, one should always be very aware of the appearance of toxic manifestations, expressed with persistence of tachycardia in spite of clinical and gasometric improvement, cardiac arrhythmias, nausea, vomiting, headache, insomnia, convulsions, encephalopathy, among others.

1.3. Anticholinergics

They are atropine-derived compounds that exert their action by blocking muscarinic receptors, in competition with acetylcholine released by vagal action, and prevent their bronchoconstrictor effect. Their therapeutic efficacy depends on the extent to which the bronchoconstrictor cholinergic reflex contributes to the total bronchospasm present and on the participation of parasympathetic v^as in bronchospastic responses which varies from person to person; moreover, it should be remembered that in asthma, the fundamental bronchoconstrictor component is the release of mediators against which anticholinergics are ineffective.

Inhaled anticholinergics achieve a lower bronchodilator effect and lower predictable clinical response than beta-2-agonists, but may provide additional bronchodilation when given in combination (salbutamol/albuterol+ipatropium bromide).

Ipratropium bromide with recommended doses of 0.25- 0.5 mg by nebulization every 20 min up to three doses, associated to salbutamol, then it should be continued every 2 h to 4 h, as needed. The onset of action is 20 minutes, with a maximum effect in 1 to 2 hours. Its collateral effects are presented with very little frequency and intensity, since the absorption of this agent is very limited, but at present its use in acute asthma in hospitalized patients has been substituted by another antagonist of prolonged action of the muscarinic receptors (LAMA), called tiotropium, which is an antagonist of prolonged action of the muscarinic receptors (LAMA), called tiotropium which is the only one approved to enhance bronchodilation in bronchial asthma since 2015, as a new indication for use in this condition, to be found in recent studies of Phase II and Phase III EC, that it improves lung function, bronchodilation and adherence to treatment in bronchial asthma, unlike the short-acting muscarinic receptor antagonists (SAMA), ipratropium bromide and oxitropium, which are no longer recommended in acute asthma, because of their short duration and weak bronchodilator effect associated with the fact that they are not selective on the M1 and M3 subtypes of the muscarinic receptors and also selectively antagonize the M3 subtypes of the muscarinic receptors. Thiotroprium, which is a LAMA, antagonizes the M1 and M3 subtypes of the muscarinic receptors with an affinity 20 times higher than ipratropium and with a longer half-life of about 35 h, used only once a day in doses of 2.5 pg/day to 5 pg/day, a greater bronchodilation is achieved.

7. Anti-inflammatory drugs. Corticosteroids

As asthma is an inflammatory disease, corticosteroids are an essential indication in the treatment of acute asthma and are a first-line drug in its treatment whether or not the patient is a regular user of oral or inhaled steroids. The consensus of most researchers and clinicians is that steroid-induced improvement of asthma attacks occurs 6 to 12 hours after steroid administration. Its basic mechanisms of action are related to its anti-inflammatory action, several mechanisms have been suggested including:

— They increase the response to beta agonists.

They reduce cell activation and recruitment. Inhibit proinflammatory cytokines (interleukin 1, interleukin 4, interleukin 13, interleukin 16, GM-CSF).
— Inhibit the release of macrophage and basophil mediators.
— Regulates Th1 cells and induces interferon alpha and interleukin 12.
— Inhibit the release of arachidonic acid metabolites of platelet-activating factor.
— They reduce the influx of inflammatory cells by inhibition of chemokines and other factors.
— Decrease the response to neuropeptides.
— IgE levels decrease.

The main effects of steroids in acute asthma access are:
— Decrease in capillary permeability.
— Reduced mucus production in the airway.
— Decreased vascular leakage of endothelial cells.
— Decrease of edema and inflammation of the airway.
— Decreased smooth muscle contraction.
— Increased surfactant.

Intravenous steroids are preferred until improvement is achieved and oral steroids are restored. Start with an initial dose of methylprednisolone (1.5 mg/kg/dose to 2 mg/kg/dose) or hydrocortisone (10 mg/kg), followed by intravenous administration of methylprednisolone (0.5 mg/kg to 1 mg/kg/6 hours) or hydrocortisone (10 mg/kg) every 4 to 6 hours. Although the initial use of a bolus of corticosteroids is widespread, no evidence has been shown to support the additional benefit of this practice. The oral route, is initiated after the first 48 h to 72 h, with prednisone (1-2mg/kg/day, in two moments of the day, in the morning 8:00am and 3:00pm, for 5 to 7 days (without exceeding 40 mg per dose) and is suspended at the end, in pediatrics there is no evidence to guide towards the progressive decrease of the dose.

Inhaled steroids have been tried in acute asthma attacks, but they are not an accepted therapy by most researchers and for this reason they are not recommended; they are more used to avoid relapses after an attack or for the treatment of prevention of acute attacks, the most used are beclomethasone, triamcinolone, budesonide, fluticasone and flunisolide.

8. Therapeutic measures in the management of crises that do not respond to conventional treatment.

8.1. Magnesium sulphate

The search for other bronchodilator agents useful in the treatment of acute asthma led to the use of magnesium sulphate. The main question is that magnesium treatment does not offer significant advantages over treatment with repeated doses of inhaled beta-2. The mechanism of action is related to the movement of calcium across the cell membrane, reduces the uptake of calcium by bronchial smooth muscle, resulting in bronchodilation. Magnesium also inhibits the release of histamine from mast cells, which decreases the response of inflammatory mediators and decreases the amount of neurotransmitters released at motor nerve terminals. It is used in doses of 25 to 75 mg/kg/dose at first 30 minutes and then every four hours. The effect of magnesium becomes evident within 2 min to 5 min after initiation of treatment, but disappears when the infusion is discontinued. It is considered a safe drug, with few side effects, the most important ones described are hypotension, so urinary flow should be monitored. Currently the use of magnesium sulfate remains as an optional therapy in patients with severe bronchospasm who respond incompletely to conventional treatment.

8.2. Heliox

Although used in the treatment of asthma since the 30's of the 20th century, it is only very recently that the systematic use of a mixture of oxygen (20%, 30% or 40%) and helium (60%, 70% or 80%) respectively, known as Heliox, has been recommended. It is an inert gas with no known side effects, with a lower density than ambient air, facilitates the passage of gases through partially collapsed airways and is associated with SABA treatment. It has been suggested that when administered through a mask or endotracheal tube, it decreases airway resistance, paradoxical pulse, alveolar-arterial oxygen gradient and increases peak expiratory flow, all of which may have a potential effect in decreasing respiratory muscle fatigue, providing more time for other measures to resolve bronchospasm and pulmonary insufflation. Its limitation is given because the effects are obtained only while breathing the gas and in patients who require high concentrations of oxygen should not be used. In Cuba it has not been used, but controlled multicentric studies are needed to demonstrate its true utility.

8.3. Ketamine

Ketamine is a general anesthetic agent with bronchodilator property, its effect is achieved by its action on various receptors and the inflammatory cascade that mediate bronchospasm. So^ it has that:

— Suppresses macrophage activity in its oxidative function and cytokine production.
— Interferes with inflammatory cell recruitment and cytokine production.
— Decreases the concentration of interleukin 4.

The recommended initial dose is 1 - 2 mg/kg as a bolus, followed by 1 mg/kg/hour as a continuous infusion. Its use may be effective at the initial time of intubation of a patient with severe bronchospasm or in life-threatening situations when conventional therapy has failed to achieve a clear improvement with imminent danger of death. As an adverse event it may promote increased bronchial secretions and laryngospasm, and may cause tachycardia, hypertension and delirium.

8.4. Inhaled anesthetic agents

Inhalation anesthetic agents (halothane, isoflurane, sevoflurane), have potent bronchodilator effects in asthmatic patients. Experimental evidence indicates that these drugs have a direct effect on bronchial smooth muscle mediated by actions on calcium-dependent channels, as well as a vagal modulating effect on bronchoconstrictor mechanisms. Moreover, these drugs reduce pulmonary vascular tone with a resultant decrease in pulmonary artery pressure in acute asthma. It is obvious that the use of these drugs in the intensive care unit should be performed by qualified personnel.

8.5. Venovenous extracorporeal membrane oxygenation with carbon dioxide scavenger

Anecdotal experiences have been described in exceptional cases in asthmatics who do not improve with mechanical ventilation. They are a very invasive procedure with a high risk of complications.

8.6. Future biological therapies

The most promising new treatment options for asthma are represented by biologic therapies, in particular monoclonal antibodies against selective targets. The anti-IgE monoclonal antibody (omalizumab) improves asthma control in allergic patients, reduces the use of inhaled steroids and the requirement for rescue beta-2 medication. Its role in severe acute asthma is not studied. Other drugs under study are interleukin 4/interleukin 13 antagonists, anti-interleukin 5 monoclonal antibodies, anti-interleukin 9 monoclonal antibodies, anti-tumor necrosis factor alpha monoclonal antibodies, and monoclonal antibodies against T cells. Also under investigation is the use of inhaled natural surfactants, based on the ability to produce simultaneous pulmonary capillary dilation and alveolar distensibility, followed by ciliary stimulation that achieves bronchial tree clearance. All of these potential new therapeutics for acute and chronic asthma need to be further refined to phase III and IV CEs before they can be established as standard clinical practice with precise indications.

9. Ventilatory treatment

9.1. Non-invasive ventilation

Non-invasive mechanical ventilation (NIV) refers to any type of ventilation without the presence of an intratracheal tube. In pediatrics it is becoming more and more widely used, there are more and more pediatric NIV ventilators on the market, as well as interfaces adapted to different ages. NIV is a treatment option and can reduce the need for intubation in a selected group of patients with severe asthma and hypercapnia, the results in the treatment of severe bronchial asthma crisis are successful although it should be instituted in the early stages of the crisis. The aim of non-invasive ventilation is to reduce the work of breathing and avoid muscle fatigue while bronchodilator treatment is administered. As for the patient's evolution, if there is improvement, the removal of the mask or the reduction of the pressure support should be initiated after a prudent period of time has elapsed. If the patient does not improve, the necessary elements for intubation should be available and invasive mechanical ventilation should be started.

9.1.1 CPAP: Known as continuous pressure in the airways, its physiology is to increase the functional residual capacity that keeps it open with the minimum constant pressure, which avoids ateletrauma and barotrauma, increases pulmonary distensibility, decreases the work of breathing, improves the ventilation/perfusion ratio and decreases the collapse of the airway during expiration. It is indicated in childhood asthma in the early stages where there is no deterioration of the level of consciousness but it is necessary to maintain continuous monitoring of the patient at all times to warn the failure or success of this resource. There are two types of CPAP generator systems, constant flow

and variable flow. It is necessary to program the ventilator well and check for leaks and interfaces.
- Flow is prefixed, 3 X minute volume (tidal volume X respiratory rate).
- Inspired oxygen fraction below 60%.
- To preset CPAP (relates to positive end-expiratory pressure (peep) on continuous flow ventilators and positive expiratory pressure (epap) on invasive ventilation ventilators.
a) Start with low values of 4 cmH2O.
b) It is increased by 2 in 2 cmH2O, according to need and tolerance.
c) CPAP greater than 10 cmH2O is not well tolerated in children.

If the patient does not feel comfortable, gentle sedoanalgesia with midazolam (0.1mg/kg/dose) and fentanyl (1mcg/kg/dose) can be used.

The effectiveness of this strategy is tested after an evaluation within an hour of initiation, where:
- The SpO2/inspired oxygen fraction ratio is greater than 200 mmHg with CPAP greater than 5 cmH2O.
-. Decreases the work of breathing.
- Decreases heart and respiratory rate.
- Patient comfort.
- Improves color and clarity without deterioration of the level of consciousness.

It is considered a failure when:
- Ph less than 7.20.
- Carbon dioxide pressure greater than 60 mmHg.
- It is necessary to increase the inspired fraction of oxygen more than 60% with CPAP of 10 cmH2O.
- SpO2 less than 90% with inspired oxygen fraction of 60% and CPAP of 10 cmH2O.
- Increased work of breathing.
- Decreased level of consciousness.

9.1.2 High inspiratory flow oxygen therapy

In recent years, high-flow oxygen therapy has been described as a useful alternative to conventional oxygen therapy in patients with acute respiratory failure with preserved respiratory effort. High flow oxygen therapy allows the administration of a warm and humid gas flow up to 60 L/min through nasal cannulas, minimizing the adverse effects on the nasopharyngeal structures, with which a rapid improvement of the symptoms is obtained due to different mechanisms such as a reduction of the resistance of the upper airway, decreases the dead space in the nasopharynx, increases lung compliance, changes in the circulating volume and also generates a certain degree of positive intrapulmonary pressure. Moreover, all this is achieved together with a better tolerance and comfort for the patient. However, the experience in pediatrics needs more research and there are no clinical guidelines that establish recommendations for its widespread use. It can delay the use of NIV although 40% of those who use it require escalation to NIV. Programmed at 1-2 L/kg/minute. Temperature of 34 to 38^0C. 95% relative humidity. As shown in table 6.

Table 6. High inspiratory flow oxygen therapy schedule

	NB <4 kg	Neonate >4kg	6-1 0kg	10-20 kg	20-40kg	>40kg
Start (lpm) FIO2	1L/kg	6 L 40%	8 L 40%	10 L 40%	15L 40%	15L 40%
Maximum (lpm)	max 5-8L	2L/kg/min (max 8L)	2L/kg/min (max 15L)	20	25	40

They are a good answer:
- Decrease in heart rate and respiratory rate 60 minutes after onset.
- Decreased need to increase the inspired oxygen fraction.
- Improvement of the respiratory work.

To identify non-responders we have 90 minutes of surveillance and that manifest the following characteristics clocas and hemogasometric:
- Carbon dioxide pressure greater than 50 mmHg.
- Ph less than 7.30.
- No improvement in heart and respiratory rate.
- Low respiratory rate.
- Thoracic-abdominal dissociation.
- No decrease in inspired fractional oxygen requirements in the first two hours.

9.2. Invasive mechanical ventilation

9.2.1. Principles of mechanical ventilation

Airway obstruction causes a series of unfavourable alterations including mechanical inefficiency of the inspiratory muscles, decreased lung compliance and increased inspiratory load due to the presence of positive self-pressure at the end of expiration.

The progressive insufflation mechanism reaches a point where the entire

inspired volume is exhaled before the next inhalation. This adaptive mechanism fails in very severe cases, and the hyperinflation required to maintain normocapnia causes progressive muscular exhaustion, respiratory failure and increasing hypoxemia. In these cases it is necessary to resort to mechanical ventilation and its objectives are very clear:
— Maintain an adequate supply of oxygen to the vital organs.
— Maintain pH in non-harmful ranges.
— Minimization of the risk of barotrauma.

The pediatric patient with severe airflow obstruction is one of the most difficult challenges of mechanical ventilation. The delivery of tidal volumes and normal minute volumes by the ventilator can cause severe gas trapping and hemodynamic compromise. This phenomenon is proportional to the minute volume and within seconds causes a significant drop in blood pressure and increase in heart rate. In this way, dynamic hyperinflation is perpetuated, because the obstruction to airflow prevents complete expiration, which when interrupted by the next inhalation traps gas successively and the exhaled tidal volume is lower in each respiratory cycle which favors air trapping.

Barotrauma is a significant cause of morbidity and mortality affecting at least 6% of ventilated patients with asthma and its incidence is related to the severity of entrapment in the collapsed or occluded airway after expiration and the regional heterogeneity of airflow distribution. In summary, the ventilatory strategy is aimed at avoiding dynamic hyperinflation, air trapping with the occurrence of barotrauma and hemodynamic compromise.

To achieve these goals, a versatile mechanical ventilator is selected with monitoring systems in its programming to evaluate variables related to dynamic hyperinflation and positive end-expiratory self-pressure. Ventilation strategies that minimize dynamic hyperinflation, use a low tidal volume and prolonged expiratory time by increasing inspiratory flow and decreasing respiratory rate should be used. The following are some of the mistakes that are made in the treatment of asthmatic patients on mechanical ventilation: - Delayed intubation.
— Focus the programming of mechanical ventilation on the correction of hypercapnia.
— Downplaying the importance of respiratory mechanics monitoring.
— Insufficient volume replacement in the face of arterial hypotension.
— Do not use full pharmacological treatment.

— Discard the inhalation route for the administration of bronchodilators.
— Administer muscle relaxants when it is not essential.
— Prolong the period of mechanical ventilation.

9.2.2. Endotracheal intubation and starting mechanical ventilation

Endotracheal intubation and mechanical ventilation can be life-saving therapies when implemented at the right time, but it is not recommended to abuse these indications as they may increase morbidity and in certain conditions mortality. The decision to intubate a patient and initiate mechanical ventilation is based on clinical criteria, its absolute indications being respiratory arrest and marked depression of consciousness due to intense respiratory acidosis. On the other hand, no two asthmatic patients are alike and each one needs to be personalized when evaluating these indications, so that a guideline can be used when deciding on this procedure: 9.2.2.1:

- Cardiorespiratory arrest or imminent cardiac arrest.
- Hypoxemia (arterial oxygen pressure less than 60 mmHg or arterial oxygen pressure/inspiratory oxygen fraction less than 200 or inspired oxygen fraction less than 235), hypercapnia (arterial carbon dioxide pressure greater than 65 mmHg) and severe respiratory acidosis with marked depression of consciousness.

9.2.2.2. Endotracheal intubation according to clinical judgment:

- Inability of conservative treatment to correct hypoxemia, hypercapnia, acidosis and progressive somnolence.
- Unfavourable evolution during treatment with non-invasive mechanical ventilation.
- Moderate sensory depression or marked excitement.
- Hemodynamic instability or arrhythmias.
- Hypoxemia refractory to oxygen administration.
- Progressive acidosis or very important acidemia.
- Intolerable dyspnea.
- Clinical signs of diaphragmatic dysfunction (paradoxical breathing) or muscular exhaustion (disappearance of the paradoxical pulse).
- Silent thorax (disappearance of wheezing).
- Cyanosis.

Intubation can be difficult in pediatric asthmatic patients and worsen bronchospasm by triggering vagal reflexes due to excessive manipulation of

the airway, so it should be performed by an experienced physician to decrease the incidence of complications:
— Laryngospasm/bronchospasm.
— Inability to intubate/ esophageal intubation.
— Bronchoaspiration.
— Injuries to oral cavity, teeth, pharynx, glottis or esophagus.
— Intubation of the right truncus bronchus:
- Pneumothorax.
- Delayed procedure hypoxemia/cardiac arrest.

It is recommended to use a rapid sequence intubation technique, prior analgesia/sedation and with the addition of neuromuscular blocking agents. Oral intubation with a larger diameter tube, according to age (4 + (age in years/4)) is recommended to facilitate suctioning of respiratory secretions and decrease airway resistance and positive self-pressure at the end of expiration. The position of the endotracheal tube should be assessed by X-ray to avoid selectivity of ventilation. Hypotension may occur after intubation, attributable to multiple factors: loss of vascular tone (due to sedation and loss of sympathetic activity), hypovolaemia (due to large insensible losses and decreased fluid intake) and to initial "overzealous" ventilation with a self-inflating bag, which may lead to damaging levels of hyperinflation.

9.2.3. Ventilation strategy

The approach to mechanical ventilation in severe asthma has varied in recent years. Since the emergence of protective ventilation techniques these have become the preferred approach to asthmatic ventilation and although in practice there is no real possibility of applying a single scheme, assurance of ventilatory goals must be achieved in a progressive manner so as not to cause lung damage. Currently the recommended technique to avoid excessive airway pressure and reduce dynamic hyperinflation is "controlled hypoventilation with permissive hypercapnia". It consists of minimizing insufflation pressure using low levels of minute ventilation associated with hypercapnia and respiratory acidosis:

- Objective: to reduce dynamic hyperinflation.
- Strategy: controlled hypoventilation with permissive hypercapnia.
- Use:
- Low tidal volume.

- Relatively low respiratory rate.
- Prolonged expiratory time.
- High inspiratory flow.
- Initial fan setting:
- Tidal volume: 4 mL/kg to 6 mL/kg.
- Respiratory rate: low according to age
- Inspiratory time: 0.8 s to 1.0 s.
- Expiratory time: greater than 4 sec.

- Maintain:
- Plateau pressure: less than or equal to 30 cmH2O.
- Peak pressure not to exceed 35 cmH2O
- I:E ratio: 1:3.
- Inspiratory oxygen fraction below 60% to allow me an SpO2 of 92%.
- Carbon dioxide partial pressure: less than or equal to 90 mmHg.
- pH: less than or equal to 7.20.

- Ventilatory mode: PCV, VCV, PSV, SIMV, VCRP, BIPAP.

The most effective way to increase expiratory time is to decrease the respiratory frequency, although its effectiveness is limited when the minute volume is low, another contribution can be achieved by decreasing the inspiratory time with a given respiratory frequency. Although it is advisable to avoid a prolonged inspiratory time, its duration should not be less than 0.75 s so as not to make intrapulmonary gas distribution even more difficult. The inspiratory flow rate should be adequate to obtain the desired inspiratory time and programmed tidal volume.

A high inspiratory flow should be used, with a decelerating waveform. This allows a complete or almost complete exhalation of the inspired volume and limits hyperinflation.

Caution should be exercised in the programming and interpretation of the inspiratory/expiratory ratio, as it can be misleading: an adequate inspiratory/expiratory ratio (1:3) may be obtained with an inspiratory time that is too short and an expiratory time that is insufficient for the patient with obstructed flow. The initial inspired oxygen fraction should be 100%, tapered to levels that maintain an oxygen saturation of 92%, to avoid biotrauma. In most patients an inspired oxygen fraction of 30% to 50% is sufficient to maintain an arterial oxygen pressure above 60 mmHg.

These strategies may result in some degree of hypercapnia and respiratory acidosis. However, the resulting hypercapnia is well tolerated by the sedated patient and if the carbon dioxide partial pressure is maintained below 90 mmHg. However, caution should be exercised in patients with associated pulmonary hypertension. Correction with bicarbonate is not recommended unless the pH falls below 7.10.

The use of positive end-expiratory pressure in patients with severe flow obstruction during ventilation is controversial. Some authors have described the worsening of dynamic hyperinflation with the application of this technique and advise against it.

The use of positive end-expiratory pressure is of interest in a group of patients who show a response of reduced hyperinflation due to decreased expiratory resistance, with increased expiratory flow and a fall in functional residual capacity and plateau pressure when modest levels of positive end-expiratory pressure are applied (below the level of positive end-expiratory self-pressure). It is proposed that the mechanical effect of expiratory pressure can cause dilation of small bronchi and the maintenance of airway geometry, moderates the phenomenon of airway collapse and improves pulmonary emptying; this is the reason for its use, provided that the summation effect is avoided.

In accordance with this evidence, the proposed conduct is to perform a test of If positive end-expiratory pressure is applied in ascending steps of 2 cmH2O, assessing plateau pressure behavior, a moderate level of positive end-expiratory pressure can be used unless it causes an increase in plateau pressure, indicating that the flow-limiting mechanism is not present. In practice, it is never used as initial therapy, nor is it used when protective ventilation measures fail to bring the peak inspiratory pressure below 35 cmH2O.

9.2.4. Monitoring

The main parameter for monitoring dynamic hyperinflation is the monitoring of the plateau pressure and the level of positive pressure at the end of intrinsic expiration. In this regard, it is recommended to maintain a plateau pressure level of less than 32 cmH2O and a positive end-expiratory pressure level of less than 15 cmH2O. The increase in plateau pressure is an indicator of decreased distensibility, not only due to the presence of air trapping, but also due to other causes such as pneumothorax, atelectasis, selective intubation of the right mainstem bronchus and pulmonary edema.

When there is no other obvious cause of tension pneumothorax, positive end-expiratory self-pressure should be suspected after initiation of mechanical ventilation. Quantification of intrinsic positive end-expiratory pressure is a procedure that is not straightforward, but can be performed with greater accuracy in patients under sedation during mechanical ventilation by measuring trapped volume or positive end-expiratory self-pressure:

- Detection of dynamic hyperinflation:
- Persistent end-expiratory flow on the flow/time curve.
- Presence of flow at the end of the exhalation on the flow/volume curve.

In the ventilated patient, other factors related to the artificial airway and ventilator programming can also contribute to dynamic hyperinflation:

- Added flow resistance due to instrumentation:
- Narrow or obstructed endotracheal tube.
- Respirator and circuit (expiratory valve, positive pressure valve at the end of exhalation and humidity and heat exchanger).
- High respiratory minute volume:
- High tidal volume.
- Insufficient expiratory time to complete expiration.
- High respiratory rate.

When inspiratory pressure increases, the cause should be evaluated. The difference between peak and plateau pressures is increased when the inspiratory flow rate is increased or when airway resistance is increased by increased bronchospasm, respiratory secretions, endotracheal tube obstruction, and loss of humidification device patency. These increased resistances may also increase air trapping with simultaneous elevation of plateau pressure and the difference between peak and plateau pressures.

9.2.5. Ventilation weaning

Once the stage of severe airway obstruction has been overcome with the presence of evident clinical improvement, normal arterial carbon dioxide pressure levels, peak and plateau pressures at normal values and absence of positive self-pressure at the end of expiration or less than 5 cmH2O, the weaning process is started, sedation is gradually suspended, the ventilator is programmed for assisted ventilation. Once the sensorium has improved and the patient is able to collaborate, a spontaneous ventilation test is performed, which with the patient intubated adds to the asthmatic the additional difficulty imposed by the resistance of the tube, so this test should not be prolonged and an inspiratory support pressure between 5 cmH2O and 8 cmH2O should be used to overcome the resistance of the tube itself. If the patient remains alert with acceptable vital signs and good gas exchange after 60 min to 120 min of spontaneous breathing, extubation is performed. An effective strategy is the possibility of using non-invasive mechanical ventilation prophylactically during the first hours in order to train the patient towards weaning from mechanical ventilation. If respiratory failure develops, the decision to reintubate should not be delayed.

9.2.6. Complications of ventilation

Asthmatic patients on mechanical ventilation are exposed to the complications observed in the generality of ventilated patients (atelectasis and ventilator-associated pneumoma).

9.2.6.1. Arterial hypotension

It is often linked to hypovolemia, dynamic hyperinflation, the effect of sedation and regular use of muscle relaxants, should be prevented with gentle volume replacement and proper programming of ventilation, sometimes it may be necessary to use vasoactive drugs. We must rule out the presence of tension pneumothorax. Another situation, although rare, is myocardial dysfunction associated with excess circulating catecholamines.

9.2.6.2. Barotrauma

It occurs in 6% of ventilated asthmatics and is associated with the prolongation of this, the presence of subcutaneous emphysema leads us to the diagnosis, which must be confirmed by radiography. Thoracic drainage should be performed, even if the volume of the pneumothorax is small.

9.2.6.3. Atelectasis

The presence of respiratory secretions can cause the formation of mucus plugs and the appearance of atelectasis, a frequent finding in ventilated asthmatic patients. Treatment is based on adequate ventilatory management

management and aspiration of secretions by bronchial lavage by qualified personnel under strict monitoring. In more extreme cases with extensive mucus plugging, bronchoscopy may be used.

9.2.6.4. Displaced or obstructed endotracheal tube

The tube must be fixed once it has been verified by chest X-ray that it is in the correct position. Even asp the tube can slip into the right main bronchus and cause barotrauma, atelectasis, hypoxemia and hypercapnia. Both this complication and tube obstruction should be suspected if the patient's condition deteriorates sharply.

9.2.6.5. Myopaba

The use of neuromuscular blockers and especially their association with the administration of corticosteroids, favors the development of myopaba, another important detail is the prolongation of ventilation. Peripheral and respiratory muscles can be compromised, making it difficult to wean from mechanical ventilation. This has led to the recommendation that the period of muscular paralysis necessary for the patient to adapt to the ventilator should be as short as possible.

The following is a flow chart for the management of an acute severe asthma crisis in the paediatric patient.

Asthma crisis assessment

Severe crisis
- restlessness, drowsiness o confusion
- Communication inlrecortada.
- Dyspnea at rest.
- Infant who cannot eat.
- Pulmonary score scale between 7 y 9   points.
- SpO2 less than 91% by oxy met ria

Life-threatening crises
- SpO2 less than 90% associated with:
  a) Confused/Sleepy.
  b) Cianosis.
  c) IBradicardia.
  d) Paradoxical thoraco-abdominal movement
  e) Silent thorax.

+

- Continuous flow oxygen to achieve SpO2 between 94 and 98%.
- Salbutamol nebulized 0.15 mg/kg/dose, up to max.
Maximum 5mg/dose. One nebulization every 20 minutes, up to 3 in one hour, continuous nebulization may be used if the clinical situation requires it.
- Ipatropium bromide 0.25mg/dose in children under the age of
5 years y 0.5mg/dose over 5 years, nehuli
The patient should be given one nebulization every 20 minutes, up to three in one hour, together with salbutamol.
- Prednisone o prednisolone 2mg/kg/day, max 40 mg/day (administered within 1 hour of diagnosis)

-Oxi gen o in continuous flow to achieve SpO2 ma
of more than 94%.
- Salbutamol nebulized 0.15 mg/kg/dose up to max.

Maximum 5mg/dose. One nebulization every 20 minutes, up to 3 in one hour, continuous nebulization can be used if the clinical situation requires it (10 ml of 0.5% butanol salt in 140 ml of 0.9% saline solution).
- Ipatropium bromide O,25mg/dose in children under the age of
5 years y 0.5rng/dose in those over 5 years old, nebulized with salbutamol, one nebulization every 20 inl

minutes, up to three in an hour.
- Epinephrine (1mg = 1ml) 0.01 mg/kg/dose SC, max 0.4mg/dose, three doses one every 20 minutes
- Prednisone o prednisolone 2mg/kg/day. Maximum 40 mg/day (administered in the first hour of diagnosis).
- Channel a venous line y administer:
Hydrocortisone at 10mg/kg/intake dose y then every 6 hours d
Methylprednisolone 2mg/kg/entry dose y then every 6 hours.
* Aminophylline at 5mg/kg/entry dose
* Magnesium sulphate 25-75mg/kg/input dose

- Non-invasive mechanical ventilation such as CPAP or high-flow oxygen therapy.
CPAP
- Flow is prefixed, 3 X minute volume.
- Inspired oxygen fraction below 60%.
a) Start with low values of 4 cmH2O.
b) It is increased by 2 in 2 cmH2O, according to need y tolerance.
c) CPAP greater than 10 cmH2O is not well tolerated in nlhos.
Gentle sedation with midazolam (0.1mg/kg/dose) and fentanyl (1mcg/kg/dose).
High-flow oxygen therapy
* Programmed from 1-2 L/kg/minute. Temperature of 34 to 38°C. Relative humidity 95%.

	NB <4 kg	Neonate >4kg	6-1 Okg	10-20 kg	2u-40kg	>4< JKg
Start (lpm) FIO2	1L/kg	6 L 40%	8 L 40%	10 L 40%	15 L 40%	15 L 40%
Maximum (lpm)	max 5-8L	2L/kg/min (max 8L)	2L/kg/min (max 15L)	20	25	40

++

Invasive mechanical ventilation (Objective: to decrease dynamic hyperinflation y controlled hypoventilation **strategy** with allowable hypercapnia).
* Ventilatory mode: PCV, PSV, SIMV, VCV, VCRP, BIPAP.
* High inspiratory flow, Fr, tidal volume y low inspiratory time, prolonged expiratory time
* Plateau pressure: less than or equal to 30 cmH2O, peak pressure not exceeding 35 cmH2O.
* FIO2 less than 60%, PCO2 less than or equal to 90 mmHg y Ph: less than or equal to 7.20.

Bibliografía

Aaron SD, Boulet LP, Reddel HK, Gershon AS. Underdiagnosis and overdiagnosis of asthma. Am J Respir Crit Care Med. 2018; 198(8): 1012-20.

Ahmed H, Turner S. Severe asthma in children-a reviews of definitions, epidemiology, and treatments options in 2019. Pediatr Pulmonol. 2019; 54; 778-87.

Albertson TE, Bullick SW, Schivo M, Sutter ME. Spotlight on fluticasone furoate/vilanterol trifenatate for the once-daily treatment of asthma: design, development and place in therapy. Drug design, development and therapy. 2016; 10:4047-60.

Alvarez-Gutierrez FJ, Blanco M, Plaza V, Cisneros C, Garcia-Rivero JL, Padilla A, et al.; on behalf of the consensus group Foro-SEPAR. Consensus document on severe asthma in adults: actualization 2020. Open Respiratory Archives 2020, in press.

American Academy of Pediatrics. State of childhood asthma and future directions: Strategies for implementing best practices. Pediatrics. 2009; 123:S129-S214.

Beasley R, Semprini A, Mitchell EA. Risk factors for asthma: is prevention possible? Lancet. 2015; 386:1075-85.

Billington CK, Penn RB, Hall IP. β2 Agonists. In: Page CP, Barnes PJ, editors. Pharmacology and Therapeutics of Asthma and COPD. Cham: Springer International Publishing; 2017. p. 23-40.

Bossley CJ, Flemming L, Ullmann N, Gupta A, Adams A, Nagakumar P, et al. Assesment of corticosteroid response in paediatric severe asthma using a multidomain approach. J Allergy Clin Immunol. 2016; 138:413-20.

Busse WW. Definition and impact. In: Chung KF, Israel E, Gibson PG, eds. Severe Asthma (ERS Monograph). Sheffield: European Respiratory Society; 2019. pp. 115.

Bush A, Fleming L, Saglani S. Severe asthma in children. Respirology. 2017; 22: 886-97.

Bujarski, S. (2015). The Asthma COPD Overlap Syndrome (ACOS). Current Allergy and Asthma Reports, 15(3), 7. Available at: http://link.springer.com/10.1007/s11882-014-050 9-6

Castro-Rodriguez JA, Cifuentes L, Martinez FD. Predicting Asthma Using Clinical Indexes. Front Pediatr. 2019; 7: 320.

Cisneros C, Melero C, Almonacid C, Perpina M, Picado C, Martinez-Moragon E, et al. Guidelines for severe uncontrolled asthma. Arch Bronchopneumol. 2015; 51: 23546.

Chen Y, Wong GW, Li J. Environmental Exposure and Genetic Predisposition as Risk Factors for Asthma in China. Allergy Asthma Immunol Res 2016; 8:92-100.

Clark VL, Gibson PG, Genn G, Hiles SA, Pavord ID, McDonald VM, et al. Multidimensional assessment of severe asthma: A systematic review and metaanalysis. Respirology. 2017; 22: 1262-75.

Corren J. New targeted therapies for uncontrolled asthma. J Allergy Clin Immunol Pract. 2019; 7: 1394-403.

De Caen AR, Berg MD, Chameides L. Part 12: Pediatric advanced life support: 2015 American Heart Association guidelines update for cardiopulmonary resuscitation and emergency cardiovascular care. Circulation. 2015; 132(18 suppl 2):S526-S42.

De la Torre Esp^ M. Let's talk about emergencies. In: AEPap (ed.). Curso de Actualizacion Pediatria 2016. Madrid: Lua Ediciones 3.0; 2016. p. 17-24.

Essouri S, Carroll C. Pediatric Acute Lung Injury Consensus Conference G. Noninvasive support and ventilation for pediatric acute respiratory distress syndrome: proceedings from the Pediatric Acute Lung Injury Consensus Conference. Pediatr Crit Care Med 2015; 16:S102-10.

Feng M, Yang Z, Pan L, Lai X, Xian M, Huang X, et al. Associations of Early Life Exposures and Environmental Factors With Asthma Among Children in Rural and Urban Areas of Guangdong, China. Chest 2016; 149:1030-41.

Feetham L, Van Dorn A. (2017). Chronic obstructive pulmonary disease (COPD). The Lancet Respiratory Medicine, 5(1), 18-19. Available at: http://linkinghub. elsevier.com/retrieve/pii/S2213260016304428.

Fioretto JR, Ribeiro CF, Carpi MF. Comparison between noninvasive mechanical ventilation and standard oxygen therapy in children up to 3 years old with respiratory failure after extubation: a pilot prospective randomized clinical study. Pediatr Crit Care Med 2015; 16:124-30.

Frat JP, Thille AW, Mercat A, Girault C, Ragot S, Perbet S, et al. High-flow oxygen through nasal cannula in acute hypoxemic respiratory failure. N Engl J Med. 2015; 372:2185---96.

Gherasim A, Ahn D, Bernstein A. Confounders of severe asthma: diagnoses to consider when asthma symptoms persist despite optimal therapy. World Allergy organ J. 2018; 11: 29.
Pocket guide to asthma management and prevention (GINA) 2019. Available at https://ginasthma. org/wp-content/uploads/2019/07/GINA-Spanish-2019- wms.pdf.

Hekking PP, Amelink M, Wener RR, Bouvy ML, Bel EH. Comorbibities in difficult-to-control asthma. J Allergy Clin Immunol Pract. 2018; 6: 108-13.

Hekking PP, Werner RR, Amelink M, Zwinderman AH, Bouvy ML, Bel EH, et al. The prevalence of severe refractory asthma. J Allergy Clin Immunol. 2015; 135: 896-902.

Holguin F, Cardet JC, Chung KF, Diver S, Ferreira DS, Fitzpatrick A, et al. Management of severe asthma: a European Respiratory Society/American

Thoracic Society guideline. Eur Respir J. 2020; 55(1): pii:1900588.

Iramain R, Castro-Rodriguez JA, Jara A, Cardozo M, Bogado N, Morinigo R, et al. Salbutamol and ipratropium by inhalation is superior to nebulizer in children with severe acute asthma exacerbation: Randomized clinical trial. Pediatr Pulmonol. 2019; 54(4): 372-7.

Jat KR, Mathew JL. Continuous positive airway pressure (CPAP) for acute asthma in children. Cochrane Database Syst Rev 2015;1:CD010473.

Kerkhof M, Tran TN, Soriano JB, Golam S, Gibson D, Hillyer EV, et al. Healthcare resource use and costs of severe, uncontrolled eosinophilic asthma in the UK general population. Thorax. 2018; 73: 116-24.

Kew KM, Dahri K. Long-acting muscarinic antagonists (LAMA) added to combination long-acting beta2- agonists and inhaled corticosteroids (LABA/ICS) versus LABA/ICS for adults with asthma. Cochrane Database Syst Rev. 2016; (1):CD011721.

Looijmans I, Van Luijn K, Verheij T, Overdiagnosis of asthma in children in primary care: a retrospective analysis;; Br J Gen Pract 2016; 66 (644).

McCracken JL, Tripple JW, Calhoun WJ. Biologic therapy in the management of asthma. Curr Opin Allergy Clin Immunol. 2016; 16:375-82.

McGeachie MJ, Yates KP, Zhou X, Guo F, Sternberg AL, Van Natta ML, et al. Patterns of growth and decline in lung function in persistent childhood asthma. N Engl J Med. 2016; 374: 1842-52.

Miguel-Montanes R, Hajage D, Messika J, Bertrand F, Gaudry S, Rafat C, et al.

Use of high-flow nasal cannula oxygen therapy to prevent desaturation during tracheal intubation of intensive care patients with mild-to-moderate hypoxemia. Crit Care Med. 2015; 43:574---83.

Milesi C. Annals of Intensive Care 2014,

4:29.

http://www.annalsofintensivecare.com /with tent/4/1/29

Morley SL. Non-invasive ventilation in paediatric critical care. Paediatr. Respir. Rev. (2016), http:// dx.doi.doi.org/10.1016/j.prrv.2016.03.001

Nichols DG, Shaffner DH. Rogers' Textbook of Pediatric Intensive Care. 5th ed. Philadelphia: Lippincott Williams & Wilkins; 2016.

Page C, Cazzola M. Bifunctional Drugs for the Treatment of Respiratory Diseases. In: Page CP, Barnes PJ, editors. Pharmacology and Therapeutics of Asthma and COPD. Cham: Springer International Publishing; 2017. p. 197-212.

Pediatric Advanced Life Support Provider Manual. Dallas: American Heart Association, Subcommittee on Pediatric Resuscitation; 2015.
Perez de Llano LA, Villoro R, Merino M, Gomez-Neira MC, Muniz C, Hidalgo A, et al. Cost effectiveness of outpatient asthma clinic. Arch Bronchopneumol. 2016; 52: 660-1.

Phipatanakul W, Mauger DT, Sorkness ER. Effects of age and disease severity on systemic corticosteroid responses in asthma. Am J Respir Crit Care Med 2017; 195; 1439-48.

Roca O, de Acilu D, Caralt B, Sacanell J, Masclans JR, Bierth HT, el al. Humidified high flow nasal cannula supportive therapy improves outcomes in lung transplant recipients readmitted to the Intensive Care Unit because of acute respiratory failure. Transplantation. 2015; 99:1092---8.

Rodrigo GJ, Neffen H. Efficacy and safety of tiotropium in school-age children with moderate-to- severe symptomatic asthma: A systematic review. Pediatr Allergy Immunol. 2017; 28: 573-8.

Shaw KN, Bachur RG. Fleisher & Ludwig's Textbook of Pediatric Emergency Medicine. 7th ed. Philadelphia: Lippincott Williams & Wilkins; 2016.

Shupta, S.M. Donn / Seminars in Fetal & Neonatal Medicine 21 (2016) 204e211 Sotello D, Rivas M, Mulkey Z, Nugent K. High-flow nasal cannula oxygen in adult patients: A narrative review. Am J Med Sci. 2015;349:179---85.

Stephan F, Barrucand B, Petit P, Rezaiguia-Delclaux S, Medard A, Delannoy B, et al. High-flow nasal oxygen v/s noninvasive positive airway pressure in hypoxemic patients after cardiothoracic surgery: A randomized clinical trial. JAMA. 2015; 313:2331---9.

Sulaiman I, Greene G, MacHale E, Seheult J, Mokoka M, D'Arcy S, et al. A randomized clinical trial of feedback on inhaler adherence and technique in patients with severe uncontrolled asthma. Eur Respir J. 2018; 51. pii: 1701126.

Szefler SJ, Vogelberg C, Bernstein JA, Goldstein S, Mansfield L, Zaremba-Pechmann L, et al. Tiotropium Is Efficacious in 6- to 17-Year-Olds with Asthma, Independent of T2 Phenotype. J Allergy Clin Immunol Pract. 2019; 7(7): 2286-95.

Szefler SJ, Murphy K, Harper T, Boner A, Laki I, Engel M, et al. A phase III randomized controlled trial of tiotropium add-on therapy in children with severe symptomatic asthma. The Journal of allergy and clinical immunology. 2017.

Tay TR, Lee J, Radhakrishna N, Hore-Lacy F, Stirling R, Hoy R, et al. A structured aprroach to specialistreferred difficult asthma patients improves control of comorbidities and enhances asthma outcomes. J Allergy Clin Imunol Pract. 2017; 5: 956-64.

Verkleij M, Beelen A, van Ewijk BE, Geenen R. Multidisciplinary treatment in children with problematic severe asthma: a prospective evaluation. Pediatr Pulmonol 2017; 52: 588-97.

Vrijlandt E, El Azzi G, Vandewalker M, Rupp N, Harper T, Graham L, et al. Safety and efficacy of tiotropium in children aged 1-5 years with persistent asthmatic symptoms: a randomised, double-blind, placebo- controlled trial. Lancet Respir Med. 2018; 6: 127-37.

Wells M, Goldstein LN, Bentley A. The accuracy of emergency weight estimation systems in children-a systematic review and meta-analysis. Int J Emerg Med. 2017; 10:29.

Yosihara S, Fukuda H, Tamura M, Arisaka O, Ikeda M, Fukuda N, et al. Efficacy and safety of salmeterol/ fluticasone combination therapy in infants and preschool children with asthma insufficiently controlled by inhaled corticosteroids. Drug Res (Sttutg.). 2016; 66: 371-6.

Chapter 7
When food allergy is not the first diagnostic option
Author: Dr. Raul Alberto Rojas Galarza

Introduction

In the United States of America (USA), between 1997 and 2007, the prevalence of food allergy increased by 18% and in the child population, an estimated 5-8% were affected. In 2013, the Centers for Disease Control and Prevention in Atlanta (USA) described food allergy as affecting 1 in 13 schoolchildren (or 2 schoolchildren per classroom). In Europe, the data are no less worrying, despite the great geographical variability of prevalence; on average, it is not less than 8% and not more than 40%, both sensitization and food allergy, at school age. In 2015, a study on the prevalence of food sensitization was published in five Latin American countries (Brazil, Chile, Colombia, Costa Rica, Mexico and Venezuela), 80% of the retrieved publications were made in patients with overt allergic disease, 60% described fish as the main food triggering allergic symptoms and 40% to APLV and described the prevalence of food sensitization between 30 and 80% of allergic patients and between 15 to 35% in the study conducted in the general population.

Case scenarios

One of the first articles on cow's milk protein allergy appears in PubMed and belongs to Collis (1930). The article describes the case of a girl of 1 year and 10 months. She was evaluated before the age of one year, when she was taking milk formula twice a day and weighed 7.6 kilograms. Personal history of importance included that at 2 months of age she was replaced with breast milk formula, at 4 months of age she suffered from "eczema" and occasional "asthma attacks" and intestinal "disorders". Family history: none for the disease. In October 1929, he was hospitalized for an "attack" of eczema; he weighed almost 7.6 kilograms on admission. During the next 6 weeks, she was hospitalized with daily vomiting and diarrhea and lost almost 700 grams of weight. The eczema subsided with "palliative" measures. Upon discharge, on December 18, 1929, she was evaluated on an outpatient basis for another "eczema attack". Her skin was examined and found to be markedly hypersensitive to lactoalbumin, but not to casea; she was then 12 months old, weighed 7.59 kilograms, had rickets, no teeth, could not sit up and was covered with "eczema". Due to "hypersensitivity" to lactoalbumin, she was put on a "balanced dairy-free" diet, with "supplemental" vitamins A and D once a day. With this treatment, the patient gained 230 grams in the first fortnight and 4.14 kilograms in the following nine months. The eczema subsided, the rickets disappeared quickly, the teeth "sprouted" and the child was soon able to stand and then walk. At discharge she was quite well and free of eczema and all other symptoms. She had a dairy free diet and additional vitamin A and D supplementation afterwards.

In the 1950s, Walker (1952) describes the case of a 4-year-old boy who developed mild eczema on his hands at 2 months of age. He received breast milk from birth and at 7 months weaning was attempted. He showed immediate rejection of cow's milk, and each time he received cow's milk he developed a perioral urticarial rash and his eczema worsened. He received different forms of milk, but reacted to all of them. He continued to breastfeed until he was 15 months old, also receiving solids and orange juice. He was not given cow's milk or any other substitute. Subsequently, he was seen by a dermatologist, who thought his eczema was due to protein in his diet, so he was put on a "relatively protein-free" diet based on vegetables, fruits, cereals, orange juice and a little milk, the latter of which always caused an urticarial perioral rash. She received some meat, but, although it didn't seem to cause a reaction, she didn't like it very much. The mother discontinued her visits to the dermatologist after a few months, but still kept the child on this diet. The child was referred to the Royal Air Force Hospital at the age of 4 years because he was thought to "look malnourished" and, on questioning the mother, it was discovered that for the last few months he had been irritable and tired easily, played very little and slept ("naps") in the afternoon. Sometimes, but not often, her stools were pale and foul smelling. On anamnesis, it was found that he was sensitive to the following foods and, in addition, he showed various idiosyncrasies: 1) Fish: extremely sensitive; it was described that even the smell of fish "provoked a reaction"; 2) Milk (goat's and cow's): urticariform perioral rash; aggravation of eczema; 3) Eggs: wall appear to have a delayed action; 4) Meat: did not react, but did not like it; 5) Cereals: did not like porridge; liked bread, no reaction; 6) Cheese: did not like it. Family history: showed allergies on maternal side. Grandmother suffered from asthma, a Ua from eczema and a cousin from urticaria. Her mother herself had eczema and was very nervous. On physical examination the child was very pale, with normal height and weight for his age.

She had swollen lower eyelids and small palpable "masses" on the neck. She had marked eczema on the hands, but no skin lesions elsewhere except for cracks at the corners of the mouth. No enlargement of the liver or spleen was observed. Blood count: Hb 10.5 g; RBC 2'800,000/mL (MCV 96.4 pm2, MCHC 38.8 g/L); WBC 4800/mL (polymorphonuclear 61%, lymphocytes 35%, monocytes 4%); reticulocytes 0.5%; total plasma protein 5.25 g%. Peripheral blood smear showed macrocytes with hemoglobin.

Response to milk: The child was given fresh cow's milk under supervision. Within five minutes he developed a well marked urticariform perioral rash. Later he was given boiled milk and only a very mild rash appeared. A skin sensitivity test was performed, using pieces of lint dipped in fresh boiled milk. No reaction was observed with the boiled milk. She was offered boiled cow's milk instead of fresh milk and given "proteolyzed liver extract", folic acid and "marmite" (yeast-based "flavoring"), because of the suspicion that she might have incipient B-vitaminosis. With this treatment he improved rapidly and his last blood count, taken 10 weeks later, was as follows: Hb 12.8 g; RBC 5'150,000/mL (MCV 80 pm2, MCHC 30.5 g/L); WBC 9,500/mL (polymorphonuclear 50%, lymphocytes 35%, monocytes 6%, eosinophils 8%, basophils 1%); total plasma proteins 6.5 g%. His parents stated that he was more active than they had ever known him to be. Nearly 100 years after one of the first reports, cow's milk protein allergy is still so prevalent and so burdensome to the life of the patient who suffers from it. The problem, as in the case described, lies in the implications of a "deprivation" treatment. It is one of the best proofs that, by removing the noxa, the patient gets better; but, as in the case described, the family gave her cow's milk or other dairy products in small quantities, because this meant "aggravation" of the signs and symptoms. In conclusion: both the remedy and the disease were "ending the life" of this patient. The alternative was to give the supplements that were not provided by the deprivation of cow's milk, milk replacers and the like. Thus, the importance of close monitoring of the diagnosis of food allergy or cow's milk protein allergy and monitoring the patient's development (if pediatric) or deficiency signs (pediatric and/or adult) is a crucial part of the diagnosis and treatment of one of the most common food allergies in the world.

Diagnostic

When is the diagnosis of food allergy or cow's milk protein allergy most likely?

In no way do we intend to develop in this chapter the criteria for the diagnosis of food allergy (FA) or cow's milk protein allergy (CMPA), which is developed in detail in this book. But it is very important to agree on the most important and frequent criteria, to be able to make a diagnosis of CMPA because, as we have seen in the example of the publications, even its treatment and the lack of "compensation" of nutrients and micronutrients (minerals and vitamins) suppressed by excluding foods of dairy origin, can lead to deficiency diseases that threaten the proper development of the patient, if he/she is in pediatric age.

Definition: APLV is an immune-mediated allergic response to milk proteins. Thus, milk contains casein and serum fractions, each of which has five protein components and a person may be sensitized to one or more components within any group. Therefore, APLV is classified according to the underlying cause: 1) Immunoglobulin E (IgE)-mediated reactions are acute and often have a rapid onset. They occur up to 2 hours after ingestion of cow's milk, usually within 20 to 30 minutes and 2) Non-IgE-mediated reactions are usually delayed and not acute. They manifest themselves up to 48 hours or even 1 week after cow's milk protein ingestion. We must consider that mixed IgE and non-IgE allergic reactions involve a mixture of IgE and non-IgE responses.

A first observation regarding food allergy is that it should not be confused with food intolerance (a non-immunological reaction that can be caused by enzyme deficiencies, pharmacological agents and natural substances).

IgE-mediated allergy is suspected in patients with allergic symptoms and/or signs of anaphylaxis occurring minutes to hours after ingestion of the food. *Non-IgE* or mixed *allergy is suspected* in patients with delayed or chronic

(> 2 hours to weeks) symptoms after ingestion of the suspected food or milk.

Once the clinical suspicion has led the physician to the diagnosis, the investigation begins. *If an IgE-mediated allergy is suspected*, confirmation is made by *skin prick* test or the measurement of specific immunoglobulin E in blood (spIgE, formerly known as RAST). In the case of APLV, skin testing is ideally performed with fresh milk, as commercial extracts may be less sensitive. When allergy testing does not confirm the history, the gold standard for investigating APLV is a double-blind, placebo-controlled food 'challenge'. Practically, an open oral food challenge can be used to elicit objective and reproducible symptoms. *If a non-IgE-mediated allergy is suspected*, skin testing and sperm IgE measurement are of little use. The only reliable diagnostic test is a strict elimination diet. If symptoms do not improve in two to eight weeks, APLV is unlikely to be present and milk should be reintroduced. Improvement of symptoms on exclusion of milk, together with recurrence of symptoms on reintroduction, is a strong indication of non-IgE-mediated allergy. In a breastfed infant, cow's milk protein can be eliminated from the mother's diet on dietary advice.

And if it's not food allergy ^ What else can it be?

When the clinical manifestations of food allergy are evaluated with a high degree of certainty, a diagnosis can be made. However, it is not uncommon that there are doubts in a number of patients in whom the symptoms may be due to other diagnoses. In order of frequency, we can cite some diagnoses that may initially be considered within the possibilities that explain the clinical picture presented by the patient:

- Food intolerance: For example, intolerance to lactose (the most common) or some other food may present with signs and symptoms similar to food allergy.
- In adolescence and adulthood, some chronic gastrointestinal diseases should be ruled out:
  o   Gastroesophageal reflux disease or Crohn's disease
  o   Carcinoid syndrome
  o   Irritable bowel syndrome
  o   Celiac disease
  o   Constipation

- o Gastroenteritis
- o Ulcerative colitis
- Anatomical abnormalities: one of the most frequent, especially in the pediatric age is the Meckel's diverticulum.
- Exocrine pancreatic insufficiency
- Infections (frequent in pediatric age, such as urinary tract infection, acute otitis media).
- Scombroid poisoning (a foodborne illness that often occurs in fish such as tuna, mackerel, mahi mahi mahi, anchovies, herring, bluefish, amberjack, and marlins; these fish contain naturally high levels of histidine).
- Auriculotemporal syndrome or Frey's syndrome: appearance of redness, hyperhidrosis, or both, in the area innervated by the auriculotemporal nerve in response to a taste stimulus triggered by the ingestion of different foods. It is usually due to a lesion of the auriculotemporal nerve, although sometimes there is no traumatic antecedent.
- Metabolic disorders (galactosemia, alcohol intolerance)
- Response to a pharmacologically active component (caffeine, thiamine)
- Response to toxins (food poisoning)
- Sulfite poisoning (ingested or inhaled)
- And additionally, there are also psychological conditions (food aversion, anorexia nervosa).

Therefore, when food allergy is suspected, a detailed medical history should be taken, focusing on the probable allergy, including:

- Personal history of atopic diseases (asthma, eczema, and allergic rhinitis).
- Family history of atopic disease (asthma, eczema and allergic rhinitis) or food allergy in parents or siblings
- Details of avoided foods and the reasons for them
- The investigation should include the following:
  - o The age at which the person started symptoms
  - o The speed of onset of symptoms after contact with the food.
  - o Duration of symptoms

- - Severity of reaction
  - Frequency of occurrence
  - Location of the reaction (home, school, etc.)
  - Reproducibility of symptoms to repeated exposure
  - What foods and how much exposure causes the reaction
- Religious and cultural factors that affect the food you eat.
- Who planted the concern and I suspect food allergy.
- What allergen is suspected
- The patient's nutritional history, and in the pediatric age group, whether breastfed or formula fed and the age at weaning.
- Mother's diet, if the patient was breastfed in the pediatric age.
- Details of any previous treatment, including medication used at onset of symptoms and response to symptoms
- Any food elimination and reintroduction responses
- In the physical examination, growth and development in the pediatric age and deficiency signs in the pediatric and adult age should be considered.
- Additionally, search for signs of allergy-related comorbidities (atopic eczema, asthma and allergic rhinitis).

The following chart explains better the sequence of diagnostic approach and differential diagnosis of food allergy.

```
                    INTOLERANCIA ALIMENTARIA
                              |
           ┌──────────────────┴──────────────────┐
           ▼                                     ▼
   INTOLERANCIAS ALIMENTARIAS          INTOLERANCIAS
        FUNCIONALES                     ALIMENTARIAS
                                        ESTRUCTURALES
           |                                     ▲
     ┌─────┴─────┐                               |
     ▼           ▼                               |
  NO TÓXICAS   TÓXICAS                           |
     |           |                               |
  ┌──┴──┐        ▼                               ▼
  ▼     ▼      Efecto                        Alteración
Inmuno  No      de                            orgánica
lógica  Inmuno  toxina
(alergia) lógica
```

Food intolerance. Response range (own elaboration)

Treatment

Treatment is based on the diagnosis of the underlying disease, which is the reason for the 'differential diagnosis' of food allergy:

- Food intolerances: withdrawal or intake of minimum daily amounts of the food involved.
- Chronic diseases: medical and laboratory control of chronic diseases. Evaluate for exacerbations and alert the patient to identify referrals to avoid overtreatment or unnecessary treatment.
- Evaluate the need for endoscopic and/or surgical correction of any organic alteration.
- Evaluate for signs and symptoms of pancreatic insufficiency:
  - Gas and/or abdominal distention
  - Abdominal pain, epigastric
  - Weight loss (abnormal growth curve in the paediatric age)
  - Fatigue
  - Frequent, fetid, profuse diarrhea (steatorrhea)
- If exocrine pancreatic insufficiency is a possibility, replacement therapy with **lipase** should be given.
- Infections (urinary, otic) should be suspected in the context of fever

- without obvious respiratory focus to explain it (in pediatric age) or in referred signs and symptoms (in older children and adults).
- The prevention of scombroidosis is the correct storage of fish to prevent the proliferation of bacteria, not to transform histidine into histamine. It is important to remember that cooking such fish does not prevent the disease because it does not inactivate the histamine formed.
- In Frey's atriotemporal syndrome, it should be diagnosed to avoid unnecessary food suppression. Often, the diagnosis is "self-invulsive", therefore, unnecessary restrictions should be avoided. In adults, various treatments such as anticholinergic drugs, botulinum toxin, or surgery have been used, with variable results.
- Within metabolic disorders, the identification of the triggering agent of the "crisis" is important to perform restriction and replacement to avoid deficiency symptoms.
- Within the anamnesis, identify the substances responsible for the "crisis", which should be avoided in order to avoid triggering new episodes in the future.
- Food poisoning is often self-limiting. Beware of those with systemic or prolonged symptoms.

Bibliograffa

Alvarez Cuesta C, Rodriguez D^az E, Garrta Bernardez A, Galache Osuna C, Blanco Barrios S et al. Auriculotemporal syndrome of Frey. A case of bilateral presentation in an infant. Med Cutan Iber Lat Am 2007; 35:295-297.

Berdonces JL. Toxicity of metals and trace elements and food additives. Natura Medicatrix. 1996-1997; No 45 Winter.

Branum A, Lukacs S. Food allergy among children in the United States.

Pediatrics. 2009; Dec; 124(6):1549-55.

Caffarelli C, Baldi F, Bendandi B. et al. Cow's milk protein allergy in children: a practical guide. Italian Journal of Pediatrics. 2010; 36(5).

Centers for Disease Control and Prevention. Voluntary Guidelines for Managing Food Allergies in Schools and Early Care and Education Programs. Washington, DC: US Department of Health and Human Services; 2013.

Collis R. Milk Hypersensitivity with Eczema. Proc R Soc Med.

1930; 24(2):113-114.

Domhguez Munoz J. Physiopathology, diagnosis and treatment of exocrine pancreatic insufficiency in the patient with chronic pancreatitis. Gastroenterology and Hepatology. 2005; Vol. 28. Num. SE2. Pages 22-28.

Koletzko S, Niggemann B, Arato A. et al. Diagnostic approach and management of cow's-milk protein allergy in infants and children: ESPGHAN GI committee practical guidelines. Journal of Pediatric Gastroenterology and Nutrition. 2012; 55(2), 221229.

Ludman S, Shah N, Fox A. Managing cows' milk allergy in children. BMJ. 2013; Sep 16; 347:f5424.

Lyons S, Clausen M, Knulst A, Ballmer-Weber B, Fernandez-Rivas M, et al. Prevalence of Food Sensitization and Food Allergy in Children across Europe. J Allergy Clin Immunol Pract. 2020; Sep; 8(8):2736-2746.e9.

NICE. Food allergy in children and young people. Diagnosis and assessment of food allergy in children and young people in primary care and community settings (full guideline). 2011. Clinical guideline 116. National Institute for Health and Care Excellence. Update 2020: www.nice.org.uk/guidance/cg116 (Accessed: January 05, 2021).

Sanchez J, Sanchez A. Epidemiology of food allergy in Latin America.

Allergol Immunopathol (Madr). 2015; Mar-Apr;43(2):185-95.

Vandenplas Y, Brueton M, Dupont C. et al. Guidelines for the diagnosis and management of cow's milk protein allergy in infants. Archives of Disease in Childhood. 2007; 92(10), 902-908.

Walker WF. Milk allergy. Br Med J. 1952; 2(4780):374-375.

Zopf Y, Baenkler HW, Silbermann A, Hahn EG, Raithel M. The differential diagnosis of food intolerance. *Dtsch Arztebl Int*. 2009; 106(21):359-370.; Kurowski K, Boxer RW. Food allergies: detection and management. Am Fam Physician. 2008; Jun 15; 77(12):1678-86.

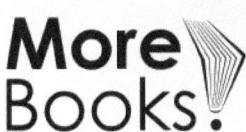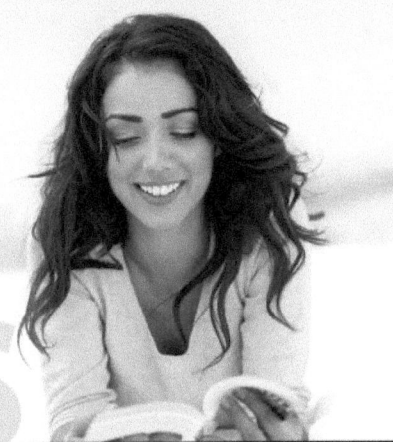

I want morebooks!

Buy your books fast and straightforward online - at one of world's fastest growing online book stores! Environmentally sound due to Print-on-Demand technologies.

Buy your books online at
www.morebooks.shop

Kaufen Sie Ihre Bücher schnell und unkompliziert online – auf einer der am schnellsten wachsenden Buchhandelsplattformen weltweit! Dank Print-On-Demand umwelt- und ressourcenschonend produziert.

Bücher schneller online kaufen
www.morebooks.shop

 info@omniscriptum.com
www.omniscriptum.com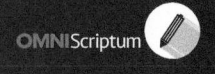

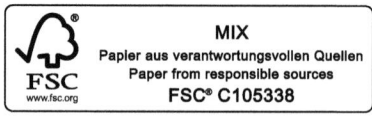

Printed by Books on Demand GmbH, Norderstedt / Germany